YOUNGER
(sexier)
YOU

YOUNGER (*sexier*) YOU

Look and Feel 15 Years Younger by Having the Best Sex of Your Life

ERIC R. BRAVERMAN, MD

Author of the *New York Times* Bestseller *Younger (Thinner) You Diet*
WITH ELLIE CAPRIA, RPA-C

RODALE

Book design by Joanna Williams

Library of Congress Cataloging-in-Publication Data

Braverman, Eric R.
    Younger (sexier) you : look and feel 15 years younger by having the best sex of your life / Eric R. Braverman.
      p.   cm.
    Includes bibliographical references.
    ISBN 978-1-60529-421-6 hardcover
    1. Sexual health. 2. Sexual intercourse. 3. Sex (Biology) 4. Health. I. Title.
  RA788.B723 2011
  613.9'5—dc22   2010030848

Distributed to the trade by Macmillan
2 4 6 8 10 9 7 5 3 1 hardcover

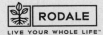

RODALE
LIVE YOUR WHOLE LIFE™

We inspire and enable people to improve their lives and the world around them.

For my children, Ari, Stevie, and Danny,
who have been my inspiration, my love, and my comfort.
Thank you for your continued faith in me.
For their mother, Dasha, who has helped them grow to become so beautiful.
And to their grandparents, Oskar and Yelena, for being powerful influences.

Disclaimer

THE INFORMATION CONTAINED in this book is intended to provide helpful and informative material on the subject addressed. It is not intended to serve as a replacement for professional medical advice. Before you begin any health care program, you should consult a health care professional regarding your specific situation. All nutrient, hormone, and medication recommendations mentioned in this book are not to be taken without the advice of a medical doctor, naturopathic physician, registered dietitian, and/or endocrine specialist.

Contents

INTRODUCTION

EVERY ASPECT OF YOUR sex life begins in the brain. The largest and most important sex organ in the body, the brain is where you experience each orgasm. It determines whether you choose multiple partners or engage in risky behaviors. It can also establish if you are a hopeless romantic or a practical partner, or determine why some people can't stop wandering and why others are never satisfied. The brain signals the rest of the body when you want to have sex, where you want to have sex, how often you want to have sex, and who you are attracted to. What's more, your understanding and appreciation of sex affects the way you love and work. It is a significant aspect of your overall happiness, your intellectual achievement, as well as your spiritual life. Without sex you cannot have a full life. And without the brain, sex is not fulfilling.

After years of research, I've found that sex is the prescription for maintaining a youthful, abundant life, and this book will show how you can use sex to become younger. By keeping an active sex life, you'll feel more vibrant, smarter, more loving, and enjoy better sleep. You'll also have a greater incentive to be healthier, fitter, and thinner. You'll learn everything you need to know about improving, enhancing, or maintaining a pleasurable sex life right now, as well as in your later years. More important, you will uncover the person you truly are—in and out of bed—and learn how you can change some of your negative behavior patterns in order to have healthier, more loving sexual relations. In short, you'll learn how to have great sex, which will lead to a healthier, more engaged life.

LIFE LESSONS LEARNED FROM SEX

Sex is greater than a mere physical release: It is the cornerstone of true intimacy and genuine relationships. It is a means for giving and receiving love, and it helps you master a whole new level of maturity. That's because dynamic sexual relationships allow the brain to think better and to love better, so that you can become a more committed, stable person who acts with integrity and honor.

To fully experience a deeper physical and emotional connection, you need to understand how the brain controls not only your sex life, but every aspect of your physical and emotional health. In this book, you'll learn how to gain sexual parity by controlling your brain chemistry. Most important, you'll learn why a diminishment in your desire for sex or a decrease in orgasmic frequency is almost always a sign of disease and aging.

If you are happy with your sex life and want to continue this level of enjoyment for the rest of your life, this book is for you. If you are unhappy with your sex life because it isn't the way it was when you were younger, I can help you reverse your aging right now so that you can return to your previous level of sexual enthusiasm. By

Every Orgasm Is a Brain Orgasm

You feel the release of orgasm in the penis, clitoris, or vagina, but the sense of calm that follows sweeps over your body and . . . your brain! Every orgasm starts, and finishes, in the brain. What's more, the brain's response during orgasm is the same for men and women, so there's no reason why women shouldn't be as sexually satisfied as men. Women who do not experience orgasm may be suffering from any number of sexual disorders, which we will go over in great detail, or they may be more guarded due to personal experiences or their interpretation of societal views. They may be stymied by an idea that "good women don't have great sex." But they can!

following this program, you can have the sex life you had—or wanted—20 years ago. And, if you were never satisfied or fulfilled by your sex life, I can teach you to make positive and lasting changes that will reward you on every level.

GET READY TO BE YOUNGER

Doctors and scientists are finding better ways to treat chronic and sudden, unexpected illnesses. So it is likely that you are going to live a long life. The real question is, what will the quality of life be throughout those years? Will you enjoy good health and an active sex life, or will you let aging and poor health slow you down?

If you've convinced yourself that older people don't have sex like they used to, or can't enjoy sex the way they used to, I'm here to tell you that you're wrong. Losing sexuality is not a normal part of aging, and neither is a decline in sexual enjoyment a foregone conclusion. My goal is for you to have a sustained sexuality that remains consistent for years to come. No matter what your age, you should be experiencing a life full of intimacy, touch, and love.

Studies show that if older adults are reasonably healthy, they can continue to have sexual relations into very old age. The best overall predictor of sexual activity later in life is the level of sexual activity in midlife. Women need regular sex to keep their natural lubrication. Men find that arousal comes more easily when sexual activity is maintained. So if you learn to revive your sex life now, you will be able to continue to enjoy sex for the rest of your life.

My medical philosophy is simple. In my New York City office at PATH Medical, the Place for Achieving Total Health, I work with a team of specialists, including Ellie Capria, RPA-C, who incorporate proven diagnostic and treatment protocols that facilitate the best of natural, conventional, and integrative evidence–based medicine. I do not practice "complementary medicine," because one does not need to complement the best that science has to offer. I do not practice "alternative medicine," because why use something alternative when you are practicing state-of-the-art medicine? Lastly, I practice a "holistic" approach that acknowledges the whole person, not just the problem, or the "hole" in the person.

My patients are blown away with the results from this program. More than 80 percent of my patients see an increase in their libidos. All of them are able to achieve better orgasm, and some achieve orgasm for the first time. Many feel that they are finally in control of their sex lives. Best of all, I find that relationships improve when couples are more sexually compatible.

I can teach you how to become 15 or 20 years younger than you are right now. Women, be ready to be sexually 30 forever. Men, be ready to be sexually 40 forever.

Women Wake Up!

The latest research is showing that the first stages of menopause begin as early as 22! This means that when you are still young, your sex life is already slowing down. It will take 20 years for your sexual self to diminish. By the time you are in full menopause, your interest in sex will be history, unless you start becoming younger now.

HOW THIS BOOK WORKS

This program offers a comprehensive plan for restoring health and reinvigorating your sex life. The Braverman Protocol offers a four-step program that includes:

- The PATH Sexual Health Checkup: early testing and identification of health and sexual problems
- Balancing brain chemistry by focusing on key food nutrients, supplements, hormonal therapies, and medications when necessary, beginning with the most natural, least invasive option until your problem is resolved
- Addressing and reversing existing illness or chronic conditions
- Creating new habits by improving diet, incorporating exercise, and focusing on self-awareness

Part I explains why maintaining your health is the most important factor for participating in—and enjoying—great sex. My unique brain-based program will help you determine your Sex Quotient, or SexQ, so you can identify the reasons why you might not be enjoying sex lately or why you might not be interested in it at all. You'll be able to determine quickly if you have a brain chemical imbalance that is causing specific symptoms or conditions throughout your body, and learn if they are affecting your sex life. You'll then learn how to boost specific brain chemicals back to normal, healthy levels, or balance them by enhancing other brain chemicals, so you can realize permanent changes to the four components of great sex: libido, arousal, stamina, and satisfaction.

Part II is specifically written for women as it presents a complete overview of how menopause causes real and lasting changes throughout the body. Menopause affects every aspect of your life, and many women find that sex can become uncomfortable, even painful. You need to know what you can do to reverse symptoms you may be experiencing so that you can continue to lead a fulfilling sexual life on every level: emotionally, physically, and even spiritually. One of the easiest ways to boost your sex life and restore your health is to return to younger levels of your body's natural hormones.

Part III is specifically written for men and the unique health concerns they have about maintaining an active and vibrant sex life. As men get older, they experience male menopause, known as andropause, and often require greater physical stimulation to attain and maintain erections. Their orgasms can also be less intense. Men will learn why it is just as important for them to maintain hormonal levels in order to feel younger in every aspect of their lives, including sex. I'll also explain the importance of preserving efficient blood flow to the brain and penis, and if drugs like Viagra, Levitra, and Cialis are necessary. You may find that there are better, more natural options that will allow you to achieve the same results.

Part IV is important for everyone to read, because it addresses particular health issues both men and women face that could affect sexual function. The fix is straightforward: To restore your health, you must restore your brain chemistry. You'll feel younger and begin to reverse illness and chronic conditions by concentrating on lifestyle changes, including exercise and focusing your diet to include specific foods, nutrient supplements, teas, and spices. Lastly, you'll learn to apply what you've learned about your own SexQ to your relationships.

Ultimately, you have the power to have the best sex of your life now, whether you are 30, 40, 50, 60, 70, or even 100. What's more, with better sex comes better health. The benefit of brain-based sexual health is undeniable: Better sex leads to younger bones, a younger heart, better memory, better sleep patterns, and better mood. A better, younger, and sexier you.

PART I

Your Sex Quotient (SexQ)

CHAPTER 1

Good Sex Is Even Better Than You Thought

IF YOU COULD make only one change in your life to improve your chances for staying young, I'd put my money on having frequent, loving sex. Every positive sexual encounter makes your brain and body younger. Everyone knows that exercise is critical to longevity. Sex is equally important.

But does sex contribute to good health or does good health make frequent, enjoyable sex possible? To my mind, the answer is both. Good sex and good health reinforce each other. Sex keeps us younger because it decreases stress, enhances intimacy, and helps form personal relationships. Lower levels of stress and increased personal relationships are clearly linked to better health. A study by the Archives of Sexual Behavior tracked sexual interest in healthy 80- to 102-year-olds. It found that 63 percent of men and 30 percent of women were still having sexual intercourse.

At the same time, studies are pointing to sexual activity as a predictor of longevity. One study has found that the frequency of orgasm for married women was protective against mortality risk. Other researchers have found a direct, positive relationship between sexuality and longevity. In another long-term study, men with a high frequency of orgasm were found to have a 50 percent lower risk of mortality than males with a low frequency of orgasm. You've got nothing to lose: Sex burns calories, and counts as a form of exercise. So as all those Nike ads say, "Just do it."

You need nutritious food to live, and you also need frequent and great orgasms to keep your brain and body in good health. One reason is that during orgasm, vital hormones are released, including the love hormone, oxytocin. Frequent sex keeps all your hormone levels up, including testosterone, estrogen, and growth hormone, which makes you younger in almost every way. So if you think you're doing yourself or your partner a favor by having sex once a month, or once a week, think again. You need lots of sex to reverse aging and achieve optimal health.

The Younger (Sexier) You goal is to never go past the sexual frequency of your forties: meaning three sexual events per week for the rest of your life, even if you live until you're 120. That should make retirement look like a lot more fun.

Younger (Sexier) You Sexual Frequency

Age 15–25	More than 1 time per day
Age 25–30	1 time per day
Age 30–40	4 times per week
Age 40–50	3 times per week
Age 50–60	Regular folks: 1–2 times per week Younger (Sexier) You: 3 times a week
Age 60–80	Regular folks: 1 time every 2 weeks Younger (Sexier) You: 3 times a week
Age 80–120	Regular folks: 0–1 time per month Younger (Sexier) You: 3 times a week

Good Sex Makes You Look Younger

Neuropsychologist Dr. David Weeks of the Royal Edinburgh Hospital found that a person's genetic makeup was 25 percent responsible for youthful looks, yet behavior accounted for 75 percent. Couples who have sex at least three times a week look more than 10 years younger than the average adult who makes love twice a week. What's more, loving couples make more of an effort to keep themselves in good shape for their partners, and they benefit from the physical and emotional effects of sexual intercourse.

HAVE THE BEST SEX OF YOUR LIFE AND GET HEALTHIER

We need to keep sexually active because sex has a function beyond procreation or recreation. Sex is like an electrical charge, and an orgasm is like rebooting your entire computer, powering up your health in multiple ways. Just take a look at men and women in their twenties and thirties: Their active sex lives enhance every aspect of their health. Here's how:

Thin, fit, and built: Sex makes you thinner, as it raises your metabolism. You're not going to drop 10 pounds every time you have sex, but studies do show that sexual activity can burn up to 200 calories. What's more, a healthy sex drive facilitates the skin's ability to manufacture vitamin D, which keeps your bones and muscles strong. Oxytocin is also known to cut appetite, as it increases the loving connection of bonding.

Better thinking: Sex helps maintain attention. Oxytocin regulates normal cognitive behaviors and functions, including aiding memory. When you're sexually alive, your brain functions faster, keeping your metabolism running high and your thinking speed quick. Most people think at a speed of 300 milliseconds plus their age. From the age of about 30 on, your brain speed slows down. But if you can maintain an active sex life, your brain will function as it did when you were younger, which means that you'll stay younger.

Emotionally stable: Sex helps to reduce anxiety and lessens cravings for drugs, alcohol, narcotics, and even food. Oxytocin lowers levels of cortisol, the hormone released when you are under stress.

Rested and content: An orgasm can help you get to sleep. Poor sleep is not only an age accelerator, but it's a sign that your brain is imbalanced. Sleep is necessary to reboot the brain so that it functions optimally during the day. Orgasm also has an antidepressant effect. A State University of New York psychology study determined that semen might reduce depression in women because prostaglandin, a hormone found in semen, when absorbed by women, can result in a modulation of women's hormones.

A healthier heart: A 2001 study from Queen's University in Belfast, Ireland, suggests that having sex three or more times a week reduced by half the risk in males of having a heart attack or stroke. Further studies showed that having sex two or more times per week seemed to have a protective effect on heart health. One Israeli study showed a statistically significant correlation between sexual dissatisfaction, frigidity, and heart disease.

Better immunity: Orgasms are thought to fight infection, increasing the number of infection-fighting cells up to 20 percent. A study released from the Institute for Advance Study of Sexuality shows that sexually active people take fewer sick days. In another study conducted at Pennsylvania's Wilkes University, students who had regular sexual activity all showed higher signs of an antibody known to fight colds and flu. For women, oxytocin serves as a natural antibiotic that can attack bacteria and decrease susceptibility to uterine infection. It also regulates prolactin secretion, an excessive amount of which can exacerbate breast cancer, brain tumors, and leukemia. Some scientists believe that sexual relations may lead to a decreased risk of cancer, because of the increased levels of oxytocin and DHEA released during sex. In men, studies have shown that a higher frequency of ejaculations is correlated with a lower incidence of prostate cancer.

Pain management: Orgasm may provide relief from pain. Some women engage in sex to relieve both menstrual cramps and migraine headaches.

Better reproductive health: A study from Planned Parenthood demonstrated that women who have sex at least once a week have higher levels of estrogen and are likely to have more regular menstrual cycles than celibate women or those who engage in less frequent sex. Studies also suggest that frequent ejaculation may increase overall levels of testosterone necessary for sperm production.

Better relationships: The hormones prolactin and oxytocin, when released during orgasm, bring out a sense of nurturing and bonding. That's why the correlation between great sex and longevity is based on the fact that you are having sex within a healthy, loving relationship, not a closed door and a magazine. Research released in the journal *Biological Psychology* indicates that prolactin released following orgasm is 400 percent greater following intercourse than masturbation.

POOR HEALTH LEADS TO POOR SEX

Both men and women can lose interest in sex as they get older. And once you lose the interest—or ability—to enjoy sex, you are accelerating the aging process even further. The question then becomes, why do we lose interest in sex, and how can we reinvigorate ourselves, and our sex life?

The answer is relatively simple. Many people believe that their loss of interest in sex is due to familial, psychological, or relationship factors. Yet I know that biological aging is primarily responsible for most sexual changes. Every day, my patients restore their lost sexual functioning, including many 70-year-olds who are hot to trot now, when they thought they were done with sex long ago. Once I reverse their aging, my patients are definitely interested in sex again. Best of all, some say that they are having their best sex ever at 50, 70, and even beyond.

According to a Duke University study, 70 percent of 68-year-old men were sexually active on a regular basis. However, this number dropped to 25 percent by age 78. With the average life span of a man in the United States being just 77 years, you have to question: Does a lack of sexual activity lead to sickness, death, or both?

In my earlier book, *Younger You,* I explained how your health is intricately connected, from the brain through the rest of the body. I show how every disease or symptom is part of the aging process. When one part of your body becomes ill, whether it is affected by a loss of memory and attention, diabetes, heart disease, or even depression, it starts an aging code, and the rest of your health will begin to cascade, pulling everything down in its path. These aging internal systems are going through "pauses," just like menopause defines diminished hormone production. These pauses are affecting your sex life and your overall health. Every disease in every organ can destroy sex. And everyone over 40 has a minimum of five hidden illnesses.

Problems like heart disease (cardiopause) and kidney failure (nephropause) can produce erectile dysfunction (ED). Diabetes (insulopause) has been shown to lessen desire, arousal, lubrication, and orgasm, because it kills nerves in the clitoris and penis, stunting the ability to experience sensuality. Menopause and andropause (the male version of menopause) are obvious contributors to sexual decline, both as a result of related physical symptoms (dryness, hot flashes, weight gain) and mental symptoms (mood swings and irritability). There are also other, more general factors that affect your sex life. I call these age accelerators because they detrimentally affect every aspect of health, making you older than your chronological age. For example, obesity affects heart muscles and blood flow, making sex more difficult. In fact, just carrying an extra 10 pounds can affect your hormone levels—including the body fat predictor leptin—which can wreak havoc on your sex life.

Any type of addiction, whether it is cigarette smoking, alcohol, drug abuse, or even gambling can also impact sexual arousal and response. Depression, stress, fatigue, and cognitive failure will also alter your sex life.

Medications May Affect Sex

Serious illness can strongly impact your sex life. On top of that, some medications that rebalance the brain or reverse illness can cause sexual dysfunction. (See chart pages 8 and 9.) Restoring your sexuality may be as easy as talking to your doctor about changing your prescription.

If You're Unhappy with Your Sex Life, You're Not Alone

According to the National Health and Social Life Survey, sexual problems afflict 43 percent of women and 31 percent of men. They can occur at any age, regardless of sexual preference. They can accompany other illnesses or chronic conditions, or can occur alone. They can be lifelong ("I've always felt this way"), acquired ("I just started feeling this way"), or situational ("I only feel this way when . . ."). The underlying cause can be mental or physical, or both.

There are dozens of different sexual disorders that men and women experience. However, they are usually categorized as one or more of the following:

- Changes in sexual energy or libido, which includes hypersexuality (excessive desire), as well as diminished desire
- Inability to become sexually aroused, both mentally and physically, including erectile dysfunction in men and vaginal dryness in women
- Inability to orgasm, including anxiety related to sexual performance, a total lack of interest, or even pain during intercourse
- Inability to properly time sexual function, including premature ejaculation

All of these disorders are real. And all of them can be reversed, treated, or even prevented. By identifying your sexual health issues, and matching them to problems you may be experiencing in both your current health and brain chemistry, you'll be able to restore your sex life. What's more, you'll be able to start getting your overall health in order just by having more sex.

I strive to use medications that treat symptoms only as a second-line therapy.

(continued on page 10)

PRESCRIBED MEDICINE	BRAND NAME	MAIN USE	POSSIBLE EFFECT ON SEXUAL FUNCTION
Antiarrhythmics			
Amiodarone Digoxin Disopyramide	Cordarone Lanoxin Norpace	Heart disease	Erectile Dysfunction (ED) Lowered libido, ED ED
Antidepressants			
MAOI antidepressants—moclobemide phenelzine	Aurorix Nardil	Depression	Decreased sex drive, impotence, delayed orgasm, ejaculatory disturbances
SSRI antidepressants—fluoxetine	Prozac	Depression	Decreased sex drive, impotence, delayed or absent orgasm, ejaculatory disturbances
Tricyclic antidepressants—amitriptyline	Endep	Depression	Decreased sex drive, impotence, delayed or absent orgasm, ejaculatory disturbances
Antiepileptics			
Carbamazepine	Tegretol	Epilepsy	Impotence
Antihypertensives			
ACE inhibitors—enalapril lisinopril	Vasotec Prinivil, Zestril	High blood pressure, heart failure	Impotence
Alpha-blockers—prazosin doxazosin	Minipress Cardura	High blood pressure, enlarged prostate	Impotence, ejaculatory disturbances
Beta-blockers—atenolol propranolol timolol eye drops	Tenormin Inderal Blocadren Timoptic	High blood pressure, angina, glaucoma	Impotence
Calcium channel blockers—verapamil nicardipine nifedipine	Calan, Isoptin, Verelan Cardene Adalat	High blood pressure, angina	Impotence
Clonidine	Catapres	High blood pressure	Impotence, decreased sex drive, ejaculatory failure or delay
Methyldopa	Aldomet	High blood pressure	Impotence, decreased sex drive, ejaculatory failure

PRESCRIBED MEDICINE	BRAND NAME	MAIN USE	POSSIBLE EFFECT ON SEXUAL FUNCTION
Thiazide diuretics— bendroflumethiazide	Corzide	High blood pressure	Impotence
Antipsychotics			
Phenothiazine— chlorpromazine thioridazine	Thorazine Mellaril	Psychotic illness	Ejaculatory disturbances, decreased sex drive, impotence
Risperidone	Risperdal	Psychotic illness	Impotence, ejaculatory disturbances
Cholesterol-Lowering Medicines			
Fibrates— clofibrate gemfibrozil	Atromid-S Lopid	High cholesterol	Impotence
Statins—simvastatin	Zocor	High cholesterol	Impotence
Other			
Benzodiazepines	Xanax	Anxiety and insomnia	Decreased sex drive
Cimetidine	Tagamet	Peptic ulcers, acid reflux disease	Decreased sex drive, impotence
Cyproterone acetate	Cyprostat	Prostate cancer	Decreased libido, impotence, reduced volume of ejaculation
Disulfiram	Antabuse	Alcohol withdrawal	Decreased sex drive
Finasteride	Proscar	Enlarged prostate	Impotence, decreased sex drive, ejaculation disorders, reduced volume of ejaculation
Metoclopramide	Reglan	Nausea and vomiting	Decreased sex drive, impotence
Omeprazole	Prilosec	Peptic ulcers, acid reflux disease	Impotence
Opioid painkillers— morphine	Astramorph	Severe pain	Decreased sex drive, impotence
Prochlorperazine	Compazine	Nausea and vomiting	Impotence
Propantheline	Pro-Banthine	Gut spasm	Impotence
Spironolactone	Aldactone	Heart failure, fluid retention	Impotence, decreased sex drive

My primary course of action is to treat the underlying diseases that are contributing to sexual dysfunction. This can include losing weight, resolving depression, and balancing your brain chemistry for total body health. If you take care of your whole body first with a brain-based program, you are likely to see the sexually enhancing results that you are looking for.

Generally speaking, my patients follow a regimen that starts with the least invasive, most natural therapies. I believe that lifestyle changes, including a diet focused on foods and nutrients that increase brain chemistry, are the first steps to restoring health. Next come bioidentical hormones, because they are integral to reversing aging on every level, including sex. Lastly, and only when necessary, I prescribe medications, which are carefully chosen to enhance multiple areas of health at once.

THE BEST FOODS TO EAT FOR GREAT SEX

Before we begin to link nutrients to brain chemistry, there are specific foods that can be prescribed to give you a sexual boost:

Food and Sexual Mythology

Foods like bananas, cucumbers, asparagus, ginseng, mandrake, and carrots are considered aphrodisiacs in many parts of the world simply for their phallic shape. The Aztecs used the word for "testicle" when they named the avocado. While these food facts are fun, they are not necessarily going to change your evening activities.

Asparagus is rich in vitamin E, which stimulates the hormone production necessary for a more active sex life.

Bananas contain bromelain enzyme, which is thought to improve male libido. They are also a good source of potassium and riboflavin, which increases overall energy levels.

Cabbage helps to increase circulation and elimination, stimulating sexual energy.

Celery contains androsterone, an odorless male hormone that is known to turn women on.

Damiana (wild yam) contains chemicals that increase sensitivity to the genitals. It is also thought to open the mind to erotic dreams. Some yams are thought to contain DHEA.

Figs are thought to increase libido and improve sexual stamina, because they are high in amino acids, the building blocks of protein.

Oysters are high in zinc, a mineral necessary for the production of testosterone. Oysters also contain dopamine itself. However, they are loaded with PCBs and mercury, so limit your consumption.

Sea vegetables like kelp, dulse, and nori contain calcium, iodine, and iron, which are all known to strengthen your libido.

APHRODISIACS TO AVOID

Ambergris: The gray, waxy secretion found in the digestive tract of sperm whales is thought to increase the concentration of hormones, particularly testosterone.

Sex Links the Brain to the Body

Let's start by understanding exactly what happens to your brain and body when you have sex. Clinically speaking, sex is the exact intersection between the physical and the emotional, both of which are controlled by your unique brain chemistry. A sexual thought, a touch, or a visual signal from one person to another causes the brain to experience erotic desire, and to release certain brain chemicals. The creative areas of the brain are stimulated to create instantaneous sexual fantasies, which in turn enable the participants to share an intimate connection. At the same time, brain chemistry activates the autonomic nervous system, causing the participants to experience physical responses. The skin becomes more sensitive, breathing and heart rate become more rapid, and blood circulation to the genitals increases.

As physical and mental stimulation increases, the physical response intensifies, causing lubrication and swelling. A woman's vaginal opening narrows and the labia swell while the clitoris pulls in toward the pubic bone. Men will experience an erection. These physical changes continue through orgasm, after which the penis returns to its normal size and shape, called detumescence, and the vagina shrinks as well. Following orgasm is resolution, during which men and women both experience a feeling of satisfaction and relaxation.

Though it is still used in some Arab countries, it is illegal in the United States.

Kissing bugs: Eating live beetles called triatomids is a long-standing practice in Southeast Asia and Mexico. These bugs are dangerous and should be avoided.

Spanish fly (cantharidin): Although it has been around for more than 1,000 years, Spanish fly is illegal in the United States. On the plus side, it causes increased blood flow to the genitals, giving the person taking it a feeling of "excitement." However, it is made from the dried body of the blister beetle, which causes blisters of the skin and irritation of the urinary tract.

YOUR SEXUAL ADVENTURE BEGINS RIGHT NOW

In the next chapter you'll learn how your current brain health is determining your sexual quotient: the particular way you perceive sex and its role in your life, including what excites and arouses you. Your SexQ is actually like DNA, a deeply embedded fingerprint that is absolutely unique to you.

However, unlike DNA, you can change your SexQ. Lots of men are born playboys, and lots of women are naturally promiscuous or sexually dominant. If your current sex life is not bringing you lasting happiness, you can reprogram your SexQ to help you become more fulfilled. Changing your SexQ is about growth, a growth that helps you become more confident in your ability to share the excitement of sex with a partner. It will allow you to experience your sexuality on a whole new level.

Refusing to take a close look at your SexQ, or to make adjustments or refinements when things aren't working as you'd like, will not help you become younger or sexier. Don't dismiss sexual behaviors that are unfamiliar or intimidating because you are embarrassed to embrace change. Instead, uncover your current SexQ so that the real conversation about improving your sex life can begin.

Start by thinking about the purpose of sex. For example, do you think that sex is all about procreation? Well, most people begin to lose their ability to procreate pretty early in life: after age 40 for women and 50 for men. So if you're categorizing sex as an activity that's only suited for procreation, you may have a good 30 to 50 years of long nights ahead of you.

Is sex romance? Actually, romance is just one small part of sex. The spark of romance rarely endures throughout the course of a marriage, but a good sexual relationship can continue indefinitely. When there is a strong sexual connection, those powerful, romantic feelings eventually mature into a deep, loving attachment.

Do you think sex is synonymous with commitment? It's not an obligation or prayerful commitment, because in that way it squashes your creativity, spontaneity, and your emotions: It just gets dull. And once you're bored of sex, then your entire relationship becomes just another perfunctory ritual. Instead, sex can be a new beginning every time.

Is sex purely for recreation? If you think that sex is just about fun, you're likely to engage in risky or even unhealthy sexual activity. You might become sexually indiscriminate, forget to use protection, become

accidentally pregnant, or get HIV or some other sexually transmitted disease. Sex is more than pleasure: It is the primary connection between two human beings. It is the chance for two people to comfort each other in a world in which we are all essentially alone.

Great sex is really all of these perspectives put together. Younger (Sexier) You means creating sexuality that is romantic, intimate, stable, and restful, all at the same time. My goal is to get you thinking and feeling about sex in the most balanced way: to incorporate each of these factors into your life, so that you have a realistic set of sexual expectations and a more mature outlook.

Get Over Yourself and Get Sexier

Our collective cultural bias has let us get away with feeling uncomfortable or embarrassed about sex, creating a completely dysfunctional SexQ. Most people are living with lies about their sex lives. You may be lying to your partner about what you really want or what you are willing to give. Yet as you've seen from this chapter, if you have bought into the myth that "good girls don't have passionate sex," only you and your health will suffer. So if you believe that you don't need to satisfy yourself or your spouse in your forties or fifties because your relationship is past that phase, think again. If you're not worried about your marriage, you should be worrying about your health.

I also find that women are more likely than men to deceive themselves about changes in their sexuality. Men come to my office with the primary complaint that their sex life isn't what it used to be, but women tend to couch the issue within the context of something else: another ache or pain, weight gain, or another complaint that falls under the category of general aging. Because of this, I find that women are not treating their sexual disorders, and as a result their marriages are suffering. They're staying committed to their Disney fantasy about romance but are not really recognizing that their lagging sexuality is a sign of an even greater health problem. Women's loss of sex drive is part and parcel of accumulating illnesses.

To my mind, maintaining a vibrant, vital sex life is an obligation you have to yourself first and your partner second. When we say that relationships are "for better or for worse," we take on the responsibility of maintaining an active sex life. So if you're having less than two or three sex acts per week, you're neglecting your obligations to yourself, to your body and brain health, and to your spouse.

In any relationship, couples may temporarily fall out of sexual parity, and the orgasm ratio—or even the desire for sex—falls. However, if you want to stay together, it's important to match each other sexually. A failure in your sex life is not an emotional failure, it's a physical one, and when it's not functioning well, you need to fix it. I promise that you can create another sexuality and keep it so you can keep up with your spouse or partner.

The goal of this book is to help both men and women gain the freedom to have the most full, intimate sex lives. I want to instill cultural changes as well as hormonal and brain chemical changes, because great sex is not only good for relationships, it's good for your overall health.

CHAPTER 2

Good Sex Is . . . All in Your Head

THE BRAIN IS like a supercomputer: It's composed of 10 billion electrical circuits that are managing every detail of your life, from your health to your happiness. But even the best computers freeze up or break down. Luckily, you have the ability to reboot your computer and clear out your electronic memory with one simple act: an orgasm. There are two ways to reboot your brain—by turning it on (as you do when you're exercising) or turning it off (as you do when you are relaxing). The beauty of orgasm is that it reboots your brain both ways at the same time.

The brain's structure, its relationship to the rest of the body, and the brain chemicals and hormones it produces all play a pivotal role in sexual activity, desire, and performance. Understanding how these factors work, and how they influence you, is the next step to becoming younger and sexier.

YOUR MOST IMPORTANT SEX ORGAN IS YOUR BRAIN

When your brain is working right, you can be a thoughtful, patient lover; you can be playful and creative, romantic or boldly aggressive, and completely committed to your partner. When the brain isn't at its peak, you will be impulsive, distracted, unfaithful, bored, turned off, or worse, feel physical pain. Healthy brain function will bring you more loving and sexual relationships, while bad brain function is connected to anger, less sex, and higher divorce rates.

Your brain—along with everything else in your body—changes as you age. And as the brain goes, so goes the rest of the body. But if you can learn to take care of your brain, it can remain active and healthy throughout your life. And if your brain is active, so is your sex life, which in turn makes you look and feel younger.

The brain is divided into three parts: the cerebrum, the brain stem, and the cerebellum. The brain stem connects the brain to the rest of the body with hundreds of nerves that branch out from your spinal column (aka the nervous system). The cerebrum is divided into two equal parts called hemispheres, which are linked by a thick band of nerve fibers called the corpus callosum. These hemispheres, as well as the cerebellum, have designated areas called lobes. Each lobe instructs your body to perform a unique function. They control automatic processes, such as digestion, and manage your internal systems. They also respond to involuntary functions, like sexual attraction, and instruct the body on how to handle the situation.

Your brain is like the circuit box in your home. When you want to turn a light on, you simply plug in a lamp and the electricity transfers from the circuit box into the lamp. In much the same way, the brain generates and sends electric currents throughout your body, fueling your internal systems and coordinating your health. These currents are transported by way of the nervous system, along with brain chemicals that regulate how this electricity is transferred.

Sexual function is part nervous system—information transmissions from the body and part cerebrum reaction from the brain. The right temporal lobe is the place in your brain that is associated with orgasms. As one writer for the *Los Angeles Times* aptly wrote, "In an orgasm orchestra, the genitalia may be the instruments, but the central nervous system is the conductor."

Sex and Brain Chemistry

There are four major brain chemical systems: the catecholamine system, the cholinergic system, the GABAergic system, and the serotonergic system. The primary brain chemicals in each of these systems respectively include:

- Dopamine
- Acetylcholine
- GABA
- Serotonin

Any type of illness in the body or in the brain can be connected to a deficiency or excess of one or more of these brain chemicals.

When your brain is working at its peak, brain chemicals are produced and dispersed at the correct levels. A decrease in sexual interest may be the first indicator that there is a problem with one of the four brain chemicals. Therefore, maintaining a younger brain by keeping these chemicals at

Sex Is Electric

An orgasm is a demonstration of how we are all electrical beings. During orgasm, you might feel goose bumps, your body hair stands up, and you feel a tingle that runs throughout your body, an electric sensation that runs from your head to the bottom of your feet. The clitoris and the penis act as lightning rods, keeping two people electrically connected through orgasm.

The electricity of great sex makes you feel physically hot, because you are experiencing an increase of total blood flow throughout the body, making you warmer and sweaty. That's why good sex or a good-looking individual is described as "hot."

	Dopamine	Acetylcholine	GABA	Serotonin
Electrical Function	Voltage (power)	Velocity (speed)	Rhythm (pace)	Synchrony (balance)
Affects Sexual Function	Desire and libido (your sexual drive)	Arousal: lubrication, tumescence, and emotional response of romance	Orgasm: the ability to orgasm and relax and bond	Resolution: the warmth, intimacy, and touch related to sex
Sex Quotient	Attraction style	Creative, infatuation style	Commitment style	Detachment or play style

the right levels is the only way to keep a younger, sexually active body, as well as a creative and loving sexual mind.

The brain is constantly creating a unique combination of these chemicals. Your genetic code plus your brain chemical makeup is exactly what makes you unique. Differences can affect your physical health, mental well-being, and personality. What's more, they combine to create a unique sex quotient, or SexQ.

If you are happy with your sex life, then your brain is most likely balanced. But if your sex style has changed dramatically, or if you realize that you are less interested in sex, your sexual partner, or any aspect of the experience, you might be suffering from a brain chemical imbalance. This might be due to illness or simply normal aging. When you can rebalance your brain, you literally turn yourself back on. A balanced brain is the only way to fully enjoy every aspect of sex now and in your later years.

The four phases of sexuality can be broken down as desire, arousal, orgasm, and resolution. Each of these phases is directly correlated to the functioning of the four primary families of brain chemicals (see table above).

Here are the basic rules:

- When you have too much dopamine, you have lots of libido but may lack stability and commitment; with too little dopamine, you may lack interest in sex.
- When you have too much acetylcholine, you can lubricate easily and feel romantic but may not be able to sustain a relationship; with too little acetylcholine, you may be dry or unable to achieve orgasm.
- When you have too much GABA, it creates tension, anxiety, and a need for perfectionism so that you can't get motivated for sex; with low GABA, you may feel too wild for your own partner.
- When you have too much serotonin, you cannot achieve orgasm; with low serotonin, men experience premature ejaculation, and women may feel a lack of intimacy or connection.

Brain Chemical Imbalances Change Your Mood and Destroy Your Sex Life

Unbalanced Dopamine • Detachment • Lack of enjoyment • Lack of energy • Fatigue	**Unbalanced GABA** • Anxiety • Fearfulness • Irritability • Rage
Unbalanced Acetylcholine • Inattention to grooming • Irrational behaviors	**Unbalanced Serotonin** • Depression • Obsessive-Compulsive behaviors

Brain Chemicals Work Together

Very few people have only one brain chemical that is unbalanced. Instead, it's more likely that there is a combination of deficits and surpluses. In fact, brain chemicals are related to each other. For example, dopamine and serotonin often work in conjunction with each other: When one is high, the other is low. So if you are strongly attracted to someone (high dopamine), you might become obsessed with that person (low serotonin), which leads to greater motivation for you to make an emotional or physical connection. When serotonin levels are high, you might have a more laid-back attitude toward your relationship and less motivation (low dopamine) to make significant changes.

Each of your brain chemicals affects the way the others work. For example, increasing the levels of one brain chemical can function like the brakes of a car to halt the effects of an excess of another chemical. This is particularly useful if you need to slow down aggressive sexual behavior caused by high dopamine levels. If you need to put the brakes on dopamine wanderlust, increasing acetylcholine adds more romance and intimacy to your current relationship. Balancing GABA puts the brakes on high dopamine by allowing you to focus on your existing commitment. And increasing serotonin will leave you more in tune with your partner's feelings, as well as his or her sexual wants and needs, instead of focusing solely on your libido.

When you hear about men like Tiger Woods or John Edwards who flagrantly go outside their marriages for sex, do you ever ask yourself why they do it? The answer is clear: They needed to apply a serotonin brake to their dopamine imbalance; without one they are indifferent to their wives' feelings. Case closed.

Date rape, murders of passion, pedophilia, and other sex crimes are more than merely bad decisions or poor judgment, or even a lack of control. They are all signs of a highly imbalanced brain.

You can retrain your brain so that sex is more balanced by doing the following:

- Redirect an excess of dopamine into your work life or exercise, or try to be less assertive within your relationships.
- Increase acetylcholine by focusing on becoming more romantic instead of purely physical.
- Increase GABA by incorporating more personal, private space for yourself to be still with thought, prayer, even meditation.
- Hold hands or caress your partner with nonsexual touch to increase serotonin.

When You've Got Your Hormones, You Moan in Ecstasy

Most people can't even say the word "hormone" without thinking of sex, and to some extent, they're right. Hormones are actually biochemical compounds that are related to the dopamine, acetylcholine, GABA, and serotonin groups. They are produced in the brain as well as other organs and glands, and they regulate specific systems in the body. Like tiny chemical messengers, hormones carry signals from one cell to another. Mostly, they're talking about sex.

A Younger (Sexier) You Influences Brain Power

Brain cell production is critical because it influences thinness, smartness, stability, restfulness, and maintenance of physical health. Without new brain cells we lose cellular volume, and we literally shrivel up all over, in the same way that a grape transforms into a raisin. Scientists used to believe that we couldn't replace lost brain cells due to aging or addiction, which led to the belief that mental capacity peaked during youth and that the best we could hope for as we aged was mild dementia and chronic illness. Yet today we know that this is not the case. While most people are losing brain cells from as early as 30 on, you don't have to.

We now know that humans have the ability to grow new brain cells throughout life, which allows the brain to remain plastic, or able to change and grow. This process is called neurogenesis and can occur when you proactively take care of the brain by raising metabolism through mental and physical exercise. By taking the steps necessary to gain new brain cells, you are improving this most central process of aging. New brain cells will not only save your memory and cognition and keep you healthier, they will save your romance and intimacy, help you sleep better, and keep you from becoming addicted. We are not destined to live out our days in the Alzheimer's ward, if we start now.

It turns out that orgasms are one way to make the brain metabolically alive, causing neurogenesis. Sex allows us to grow new brain cells because the electrical stimulation of orgasm triggers neurogenesis: It literally enlivens your brain. If you can't achieve orgasm, you are missing out on this opportunity.

The Eyes Have It

Fifty percent of the brain is dedicated to vision, so when it comes to physical attraction, you might feel it in your genitals, but your brain is really guiding your arousal. And though many are drawn to pornography, it's the wrong brain exercise. Porn isn't sex; it's a dopamine exercise that requires no effort or work. It is actually damaging to the brain because it feeds the trivial, narcissistic personality. A better brain sex exercise is to see if you can transfer your temporary lust for a beautiful young body toward a new fantasy involving your spouse.

When you were young, your hormone levels were at their peak. For example, an 18-year-old boy with high testosterone can spend the entire day thinking about his erection. People with high levels of oxytocin, estrogen, and testosterone lie in bed and cuddle all night.

But as you get older, low levels or imbalances of these hormones occur, and the ability to engage in sex becomes difficult, unsatisfying, and even painful. Without high levels of hormones, your genitals actually become smaller, and you may feel less sexy and less sexually motivated. The result is erectile dysfunction in men, and women who marginalize their sex lives. Asexuality reflects a general lack of engagement in other areas, which is one of the clinical definitions of both menopause and andropause.

In most cases, declining hormone levels are neither irreparable nor permanent. You can reverse hormone-related aging and turn your sex life back on. If you can boost the same hormones that you are losing in their most natural forms, the symptoms and conditions related to their decline will disappear, creating a younger you, full of vigorous health and a rejuvenated sex life.

Most women need more natural estrogen by the time they are 30. Most men will need testosterone by 40 or 50, and certainly by 60. Many other hormones and treatments may be necessary to completely restore your sexuality. In the next chapter you'll be able to identify which hormones you may be losing, and uncover your unique brain chemistry and your SexQ. Then you can craft a program

Men Really *Do* Think about Sex More

The hypothalamus, the part of the brain responsive to sex hormone production, is 2.5 times bigger in men than in women. This may be the reason why sexuality seems to be more dominant in male thinking: Men literally lose their heads over sex because more of their brains are impacted by sex.

unique to your needs that will not only restore your brain chemistry, increase your hormone level, and help you achieve better health, but you'll also find the keys to the active, loving sex life you always wanted.

CHAPTER 3

What's Your SexQ?

YOUR SexQ IS defined by the balance of chemicals in your brain, both by deficiencies you may have as well as surpluses. I call this the biochemistry of personality, and I find it to be one of the most fascinating aspects of brain science.

Your biochemistry not only affects your attitude toward sex and your physical capacity, but also contributes to the way you perceive your current relationship (or may be one of the reasons why you aren't in one). It helped you choose your partner to begin with and will determine the course of your relationship as you age.

When your sexuality feels broken, it may lead you to an avoidance of sex—or to pursue it in inappropriate places. You might dismiss this behavior as the result of fatigue or boredom, but I call it a scandal. We all have sex scandals when the brain is imbalanced. It might be "I haven't had sex with my husband in years," "I haven't had an orgasm in 6 months," or "I can't stop myself from having affairs and one-night stands."

Whatever it is, my program will help you understand what's broken and show you how to repair your sex life once and for all. You'll also learn how to balance your sexuality, so that you can create the sex life that you want and, more importantly, the sex life you need to be at your best, in every aspect of your life.

BRAIN MAPPING EXPOSES YOUR SexQ

My private medical practice is called PATH Medical—the Place for Achieving Total Health. It is based on the fundamental idea of early and innovative diagnostics. By using the latest technology, I can help my patients address problems relating to sex and their general health *before* real physical symptoms occur. My preventive testing can identify the earliest, tiniest internal markers that signal health problems. Because the brain and body are so intimately connected, I begin the diagnostic process with the brain.

Brain Electrical Activity Mapping, or BEAM, is one method of assessing electrical transmissions in the brain. It provides a status report of your power, or metabolism (dopamine); your brain speed (acetylcholine); your rhythm (GABA); and your balance (serotonin). The electrical impulses register as colored bursts that represent actual brain transmissions. When your brain is in harmony, the image looks like a full-spectrum rainbow, a literal "picture of health." Yet most of us are dominant in one particular brain chemical, which means that we are deficient in others. On the brain map, you can see this quite clearly when one or two colors dominate the image. From these pictures we can make intelligent decisions about which of the four primary brain chemicals needs to be addressed, and later, we can accurately assess the effectiveness of treatment.

Knowing your brain is the most important way you can monitor your health and your sexuality. We can electrically map sexuality and even predict and map your brain SexQ, and ultimately prescribe a Braverman Protocol to resolve your sexual function. What's more, we can even help match your sexual style to that of your spouse or partner.

BEAM testing should be part of every patient's comprehensive medical care. It's easy to administer, takes only about an hour to complete, is completely painless, and has no side effects.

Your Brain Medical History

There are specific health history questions pertaining to the brain that can also determine if chemical imbalances are affecting your sex life. If you have suffered from or are currently experiencing any of these issues, they may be directly related to your brain chemistry.

- Convulsions or seizures
- Depression
- Difficulty speaking
- Falls
- Frequent or recurring headaches
- Light-headedness
- Loss of balance
- Loss of consciousness
- Loss of strength
- Memory loss or confusion
- Nervousness
- Numbness or tingling sensations
- Panic attacks
- Paralysis
- Sleep problems
- Stroke
- Suicidal thoughts
- Tremors

Approximately 1.4 million Americans sustain a traumatic brain injury each year. While most people assume that brain trauma affects memory and attention, they don't realize that it can also screw up your sex life. Brain trauma can turn off the production of dozens of hormones, including testosterone and growth hormone.

Even minor whiplashes that don't cause loss of consciousness can still affect your sex hormones.

For example, Ron Duguay, the famous hockey player, recently wrote an article with me for *Sports Illustrated* to show the connection between concussion and testosterone hormone deficiency, as well as memory loss. Ron played 12 seasons in the NHL, from 1977 through 1989, all of them without a helmet. When I first met him, he told me that he had suffered from only one major concussion during his career but had had several smaller incidents. He felt that he was in great health, and he was generally happy with his life and his marriage to former supermodel Kim Alexis. Yet at 52 he was already showing signs of memory loss. Ron has always taken great care of his body, but he knew that he had to do something about his brain.

After a full battery of testing, I had Ron follow my Braverman Protocol to bring his brain back to balance. Even though he was not complaining of sexual dysfunction, his testosterone levels were low for a man of his age and his general high health level, so I prescribed a testosterone cream as well as dopamine-enhancing supplements. Within 3 weeks he told me that he was feeling noticeably different. He observed that he had more strength during his workouts, and that the recovery time between rigorous workouts had decreased. He also told me that sex seemed to improve after he'd been using the testosterone cream for just a short while.

YOUR SEXUAL TEMPERAMENT

One of the things that influences your SexQ is the way in which you express yourself. I believe that brain chemistry and psychology are intrinsically linked, and both can significantly affect sexual function. Every time I see a patient with a sexual complaint, I have to take into account not only overall health, age, and brain chemistry, but the status of the relationship, which can also be affected by the partner's own brain chemistry and chemical imbalances.

The following are quick definitions of different thinking and behavioral styles. Circle the half of each pair that best describes you. Interestingly, each of these categories,

Monogamy Can Change Your Brain

A University of California, Davis, study has established a primate model of monogamy that may be closely related to the way the human brain responds to having a mate. The study showed that male titi monkeys that were in monogamous relationships had more dopamine than lone, unpaired males. Interestingly, this brain chemistry changed when the lone males were introduced to new mates. This may mean that simply being in a loving relationship increases your dopamine levels, which in turn increases your sexual desire.

modified from the Myers-Briggs personality test, corresponds to one of the four primary brain chemicals; your answers can provide nonphysical clues to your SexQ (see table on page 197).

Extroverts vs. Introverts

E—EXTROVERTS
(HIGH DOPAMINE)

Extroverts direct their energy outward. They are very active and social, enjoy being in groups, and tend to talk before listening. Extroverts are comfortable talking about sex, as well as expressing their personal needs for sexual gratification.

I—INTROVERTS
(LOW DOPAMINE)

Introverted people require time for quiet reflection, especially if their work is socially demanding or if they are under stress or feeling anxious. Introverted individuals tightly control their thoughts, feelings, and needs and may appear aloof or distant. Introverts keep to themselves and lack interest in meeting people in order to have sex.

Intuitive vs. Sensing

N—INTUITIVE
(HIGH ACETYLCHOLINE)

Intuitives are always looking for new opportunities, new problems to solve, and new ways of doing things. They operate on their hunches, which makes them exciting companions. Their desire for change can put pressure on relationships if they actualize their fantasy life, or if they express their sexual desires too bluntly.

S—SENSING
(LOW ACETYLCHOLINE)

Sensing types value accuracy in communication and prefer to base their statements on facts. They will trust the tried-and-true ways of doing things and place a high value on tradition and experience. They are adept at managing the day-to-day details of living. Sexually they can be satisfied with same old, same old.

Judging vs. Perceiving

J—JUDGING
(HIGH GABA)

These people organize their outer worlds by means of structure, lists, and plans and need closure when working on projects before moving on to something else. Their compulsion to organize overshadows any sense of flexibility, spontaneity, or acceptance of change. Sexually they can be satisfied with routine.

P—PERCEIVING
(LOW GABA)

Perceivers are curious and love to experience new things. They adapt quickly and tend to be interested in everything. This can cause them to start many projects but lack the follow-through to actually finish them. Even though they are spontaneous, sex can be infrequent.

Feeling vs. Thinking

F—FEELING
(HIGH SEROTONIN)

Feelers have a warm, quick response to people and will try to say and do nice things. Feeling types want to be told explicitly that they are loved or cared for. Outside of relationships, they focus on human values instead of achieving goals. They fall in and out of love frequently and use sex as a way to demonstrate their bond.

T—THINKING
(LOW SEROTONIN)

Thinkers gather their information through logic and tend to make decisions based on justice and fairness. They are highly principled and often criticize others for not following the rules. Their seeming lack of empathy makes them come across as cold. Thinkers who don't attach emotion to sex lack intimacy and end up sleeping with strangers because they don't feel enough emotionally or sexually.

The blend of temperaments most likely to result in high sexuality is extroverted,

What's on Your Mind?

Sexual dysfunction may be a sign that there's too much on your mind. Feelings of anger or resentment toward your spouse can quash desire. Gender roles you may be bound to—including who initiates sex in your relationship—can also play a role, as can comparisons to previous sexual partners or sexual experiences. In fact, outside of your health, any of the following can affect your libido and your ability to become aroused.

- Family
- Friends
- Religion
- Partner relationship
- Partner's sexual function
- Personal experiences
- Psychological conditions

intuitive, judging, and feeling. But guess what? If these temperaments aren't already part of your makeup, you can cultivate them. You can work on becoming more outgoing, develop intuition, organize yourself, and connect with your feelings. You can do it chemically or by exercising your brain using a series of brain exercises I created (see Chapter 13). The bottom line is that by adjusting your temperament, you can create a new SexQ and a brand-new sex life, bringing you new intimacy, new learning, new stability, and freedom from negative or even addictive behaviors.

THE YOUNGER (SEXIER) YOU QUIZ

Even with all of the latest technologies, every experienced doctor must first rely on patient information to assess physical conditions. Because not everyone has access to my medical office or BEAM technology, I have developed a simple test that you can take in the privacy of your own home to help identify your SexQ; it is far more precise than the personality quiz you just completed. This quiz highlights your dominant SexQ and will help you identify brain chemical deficiencies that may be causing discord or dysfunction, or otherwise damaging your sex life.

While this quiz is an important step toward preserving (or resurrecting) healthy sexual function, I urge you to seek the care of a physician in terms of making conclusive decisions about your sexual health. Bloodwork as well as additional testing performed at a doctor's office can easily confirm your findings and are recommended once you have taken this quiz. A problem with your sex life may be a signal that there are other medical issues that need to be dealt with.

Many of the questions are directly related to your thoughts and feelings about sex. Some are also related to your personality as well as your overall health. Once you rebalance your brain, both your health and your sex life will improve, and you may see that these conditions related to the test disappear on their own.

Answer each question by circling either T for true or F for false. At the end of each group, record only the total number of True statements in the space provided. Answer the questions in terms of how you feel most of the time. For example, if you've had a bad night's sleep and feel tired today, answer the questions that pertain to your energy levels on average, not just today.

DOPAMINE = DOMINANT SEX DRIVE

1. My sex life began at an early age.   T / F

2. Sex without orgasm is a waste of time.   T / F

3. I like to have sex in many different positions.   T / F

4. I'm easily turned on.   T / F

5. I've cheated on my spouse.   T / F

6. I prefer to be sexually dominant.   T / F

7. My skin is incredibly sensitive to touch.   T / F

8. Next to sex, work is the most important part of my life.   T / F

9. I have been told that I'm self-centered.   T / F

10. I eat quickly.   T / F

11. I'm a smoker.   T / F

12. I've had an orgasm just thinking about sex.   T / F

13. I eat only to reenergize my body.   T / F

14. Alcohol stimulates me.   T / F

15. I have a temper.   T / F

16. I enjoy gambling.   T / F

17. Sometimes sex hurts, but I don't mind.   T / F

18. I'm hard on myself, but I'm harder on my friends and family.   T / F

19. I feel a sexual charge when my nipples are touched.   T / F

20. Coffee/caffeine has little effect on my energy levels.   T / F

Total # of T responses: _____

ACETYLCHOLINE = CREATIVE AROUSAL AND LOVEMAKING

1. Sex is the added bonus to a loving relationship.   T / F

2. I've had orgasms when I dream.   T / F

3. I long for the feeling of being in love.   T / F

4. I get turned on with role-playing games.   T / F

5. I've been told that I really "get" people.   T / F

6. I am flirtatious.   T / F

7. I am a smoker.   T / F

8. I have taken illicit drugs like mushrooms and/or LSD.   T / F

9. I have asthma; I can't breathe easily.   T / F

10. I have an eating disorder, or have had one in the past.   T / F

11. I still have plenty of lubrication for sex.   T / F

12. I have tried many alternative remedies.   T / F

13. I like to talk about what's bothering me.   T / F

14. I like reading erotic books.   T / F

15. I need a lot of love and nurturing.   T / F

16. I tend to see myself in a desirable light.   T / F

17. I have allergies.   T / F

18. I can't have sex with my spouse/partner if I'm mad or agitated.   T / F

19. I've been told that I'm often cranky.   T / F

20. I've lost muscle tone.   T / F

Total # of T responses: _____

GABA = DUTIFUL, LOVING CARETAKERS

1. I like to have sex the same time of day or night.   T / F

2. I like to have sex the same way, every time.   T / F

3. I like to take a shower after I have sex.   T / F

4. I'm loyal to my partner and would never stray.   T / F

5. Orgasms are important, but that's not all that sex is about.   T / F

6. I prefer to use condoms because they make sex cleaner.   T / F

7. I have recurring urinary infections.   T / F

8. I sense that others want to hurt me.   T / F

9. I get off by making my partner orgasm.   T / F

10. I'm anxious and blue.   T / F

11. I need alcohol to relax.   T / F

12. I have trouble climaxing and achieving orgasms.   T / F

13. I'm bored with sex.   T / F

14. I like order and tidiness.   T / F

15. Sex is just one aspect of my marriage.   T / F

16. I overeat meat and protein.   T / F

17. Sex is a chore.   T / F

18. Being in a loving relationship is the central force in my life.   T / F

19. Dinner is not complete without dessert.   T / F

20. I can only feel aroused when I smoke marijuana.   T / F

Total # of T responses: _____

SEROTONIN = SEX WITHOUT STRINGS

1. I sleep like a baby after I have great sex.   T / F

2. I'm open to trying new sexual experiences with my partner.   T / F

3. I fall in and out of love easily.   T / F

4. Sex in the morning allows me to stay relaxed all day long.   T / F

5. I frequently have erotic dreams.   T / F

6. I am a deeply sensuous person.   T / F

7. I have vast mood swings.   T / F

8. Sometimes I need to have sex twice in order to feel satisfied.   T / F

9. Nothing feels better than falling in love.   T / F

10. Sex toys are fun and mix things up for me.   T / F

11. I make lots of bad decisions.   T / F

12. I'm bored with traditional penetration.   T / F

13. I don't need to be in love in order to have sex with someone.   T / F

14. I have many frivolous relationships and sexual partners.   T / F

15. I've had many different jobs/careers.   T / F

16. It takes me a long time to have an orgasm.   T / F

17. I would have sex with my friend's spouse.   T / F

18. I rarely stick to a plan.   T / F

19. I've read the Kama Sutra.   T / F

20. I like to wear revealing clothing.   T / F

Total # of T responses: _____

Assessing Your Results

Circle the highest number. This is your SexQ, and it shows which brain chemical is dominant. The category with the lowest number is your greatest deficiency and should be addressed first. Yet any deficiency or serious dominance needs to be adjusted in order to achieve optimal health and a more balanced sex life.

There's nothing wrong with having a dominant nature. But any category with more than 10 True statements indicates that you are too dominant in that area and need to bring up the other brain chemicals in order to achieve balance. Conversely, any category with between 5 and 7 True statements is considered a minor deficiency. Any category limited to only 1 to 4 True statements is considered a major deficiency.

Frequently Asked Questions

WHY ARE THERE SO MANY QUESTIONS ABOUT MY PERSONALITY?

Too much or too little of any one chemical can dominate your personality and emotional state. And because sex is so closely linked to emotional life, these two areas need to be fully explored to expose your particular issues. Frequently, I find that when people's brain chemistries are rebalanced, their emotions can be stabilized as well. They end up getting their health under control, too, which makes them feel happier about every aspect of their lives.

In the next four chapters we'll look more closely at specific sexual disorders and personality patterns that are directly linked to deficiencies in each of the different brain chemicals. You'll find that once you balance your brain chemistry, your emotional life will become more balanced.

WHAT HAPPENS IF I HAVE MULTIPLE DEFICIENCIES?

If you've had problems with sex all your life, it's very likely you have a dopamine deficiency, as well as others. Treatment, therefore, must address multiple chemical imbalances. If you are showing moderate or major deficiencies in multiple categories, make sure to review each of the next four chapters to get a full picture of your current health. You can incorporate the specific recommendations for treating each brain chemical deficiency at the same time, tailoring the program to get the results you need. Start with your greatest deficiency. Once that improves, take the test again and see if the other deficiencies change as well. Sometimes, one small change can have a cascading effect and create better overall health.

YOUNGER (SEXIER) YOU MEDICAL QUIZ

1. Is your birth control affecting your sex life?

The birth control pill is used by more than 80 percent of American women born after 1945. However, new research indicates that "the Pill" is inhibiting more than pregnancy: It may permanently depress your sexual drive. Birth control pills are synthetic combinations of estrogen and progesterone that trick your body into thinking that it's pregnant. However, taking birth control pills has been linked to hormonal and endocrine abnormalities. First, they inhibit a woman's own production of natural androgens, including testosterone. Androgens have a direct effect on the pleasure you experience during sex.

Additionally, the Pill appears to increase the amount of sex hormone–binding globulin (SHBG) in the body. This protein binds to testosterone, preventing a woman's body from using it effectively. High levels of SHBG have been directly linked to decreased libido and sexual desire.

Long-term oral contraceptive use reduces the efficacy of oxytocin receptors, which may flatten your sex drive and block incidental, passionate sexual arousal. What's more, women don't make much of this hormone to begin with, and it's difficult to increase oxytocin without supplementation (or pregnancy). If you've been on the Pill, you probably need higher levels of oxytocin to experience strong bonding with your partner.

A January 2006 study in the *Journal of Sexual Medicine* demonstrated possible long-term effects from birth control pills on the female libido. The study found that women on the Pill showed noticeably decreased levels of sexual desire compared to those women who do not take birth control pills. It also found that women who discontinued use of the Pill continued to suffer sexual side effects. Some women find that switching to a triphasic birth control pill (which delivers differing amounts of hormones every week) interferes

Spermicides Can Be a Turnoff for Men and Women

Spermicides are not an effective form of birth control when they are used alone. Plus, there are sexual as well as physical side effects to consider.

- Spermicides must be used immediately before sex, which can negatively affect spontaneity.
- Some spermicides taste bad and can ruin the pleasure of oral sex. Try different brands to find one that you and your partner like. Or wait to apply just before penile penetration.
- Some spermicides can create numbness in either the penis or vagina, causing decreased sensitivity.
- Spermicides can cause allergic reactions or rashes on the inside of the vagina or on the penis.
- Spermicides can cause urinary tract infections, making sex painful.

much less with their sex drive than mono-phasic pills (which deliver the same amount of hormones in each dose). Bottom line: Birth control pills can cause lifelong mood disorders that will affect your sexual functioning.

Reconsider condoms: Condoms remain the best choice for preventing sexually transmitted diseases. However, many men refuse to wear them because they believe they are uncomfortable and decrease sensitivity. One study produced by Indiana University clearly showed that condoms generally "fit fine and feel comfortable." However, at clearly identifiable intersections of length and girth, comfort was an issue; there was a true relationship between penile dimensions and the perception of condom fit and feel. Fortunately, there is a wide variety of condoms in the marketplace, and through experimentation most men can find one that fits comfortably.

2. Have you had any surgical procedures that could be affecting sex?

Some procedures can enhance your sex life if the outcome is that you feel better overall. For example, studies have shown that those who have had successful surgery to reduce back pain report a significantly better sex life than those who did not have surgery. However, the same surgery can produce disturbed orgasm and genital sensation in women, and a significant disturbance of ejaculation and genital sensation in men.

Any surgical procedure will affect your brain chemistry. Anesthesia is a jolt to the brain and can directly affect both dopamine and acetylcholine levels. Check with your doctor to see if sexual dysfunction can be related to a recent surgical procedure. With that knowledge, tailor this program to meet your needs. Specifically, by boosting your dopamine, you might be able to circumvent the negative side effects from your procedure and return to a previously enjoyable sex life.

3. Have you experienced sexual trauma as an adult or as a child?

Sex therapists have come to believe that some people who suffer from sexual problems have experienced sexual trauma in their lives. This encompasses a wide range of experiences, including sexual abuse, incest, molestation, and rape (as a child or adult). These traumas can cause a wide spectrum of sexual problems, including the inability to reach orgasm, lack of interest in sex, vaginal spasms, and fear of intimacy or touching. Research indicates that about one in three women and one in seven men have been victims of sexual trauma at some point in their lives. Some survivors of sexual trauma have no memory of the actual abuse but will experience strong negative reactions during sex that they cannot explain or understand. Therapy can help survivors recover from the effects of sexual trauma by helping them develop trust, express their anger, resolve their feelings toward the offender, and overcome their fears.

GET READY TO GET SEXIER

In the next four chapters we'll examine each of the brain chemicals more closely. Don't skip to the chapters that directly relate to your results on the quiz: Read all the information in order to get the best, and fastest, results. Even if you don't feel a dopamine deficiency is the root of your sexual problems, or the test revealed that other brain chemicals may be more out of balance, I can guarantee you'll get the best results if you incorporate the lessons regarding dopamine.

In fact, each of the next four chapters has great strategies that anyone, regardless of their brain chemistry, can learn from.

Once you begin to balance your brain, you will automatically feel younger, and hopefully, sexier. Your brain will be working optimally, and along with having better sex, you may experience better moods, better memory retention, and even better sleep. These positive outcomes will affect your sex life as well: When you are thinking more clearly and feeling refreshed, as well as better about yourself, you will have a much better attitude toward sex. Most important, you'll be able to look at your relationship in a whole new, loving light.

CHAPTER 4

Dopamine Drives Sexual Desire

SEX IS TRIGGERED by dopamine and its family of chemicals, which are various forms of norepinephrine and brain amphetamines. They are your brain's natural power source, governing your metabolism, and are associated with feelings of pleasure, motivation, and concentration. According to the book *The Science of Orgasm,* dopamine and its receptors are exactly what enhance sexual behavior.

Dopamine is released from the limbic system, or the "reward" center of the brain. The central job of dopamine and its related chemicals is to keep us working—that is, engaged in activities that are necessary for survival, such as eating, having sex, and breathing. Dopamine rewards us by making us feel good as we are performing these tasks. It is also related to how we control a potential addiction, whether it is caffeine, nicotine, alcohol, food, shopping, or sex.

When your dopamine levels are high, you experience physical attraction and have the energy to take action as well as ability to perform. You'll perceive yourself as "sexy" with a strong libido. Sex for those with a high level of dopamine is gratifying because all five senses are awakened, and during orgasm you will experience an actual instantaneous release of more dopamine, which feels like a little jolt of pleasure. In fact, orgasm is the brain's reward to you for having sex.

In addition to making you feel good during sex, dopamine ensures that you'll repeat the behavior whenever possible. It does this by activating the regions of the brain that control memory. This is called the reward pathway. It signals the brain regions involved in memory and enables the brain to create the memory that sex makes you feel good. This increases the likelihood that you will want to have sex again.

When your brain is creating too much dopamine, you may feel physically hot. Your metabolism races, and you can't keep up with your hunger. Sexually, you might desire several different partners, you might need to have sex all the time, or you might crave a constant variety of positions or locations. While variety may be the spice of life, this behavior often leads to failed relationships if your partner is not equally open to new

Dopamine Sexual Archetypes

Dopamine can bring out the best and the worst in people. However, negative traits on either end of the spectrum often lessen—even vanish—when your brain chemistry is rebalanced.

Too Much: Casanova—addicted to sex and variety

Too Little: Emily Dickinson—alienated herself from sex as well as the rest of the world

ideas. I've also found that people who are too interested in variety are vulnerable to unfaithfulness and romantic disappointment. If this is your SexQ, you might have to learn to dial down your desires and your libido.

If you scored high in the dopamine section of the quiz in Chapter 3, you already have an abundance of dopamine. This means you usually have lots of energy for sex and plenty of interest as well. Your day is organized, and you look forward to spending time alone with your spouse or partner. If you are not in a relationship, you consider meeting new people an adventure, and dating comes easily. You may have a cavalier attitude toward sex because your need for it is strong. The downside of this is that sometimes your relationships are not exactly deep and meaningful, so while your sex life is great, your love life might not be all that.

When your dopamine is low, it affects your emotional stability as well as your sexual performance. Without dopamine, your sex life loses its spark. You may be too tired to have sex. And when you can rise to the occasion, you'll find that it's harder for you to get sufficiently enthusiastic.

When you are low in dopamine, two important changes occur to your sex life:

- Low dopamine—low libido or desire
- Low dopamine—low stamina or performance (weak erections for men, difficulty achieving orgasm for women)

Your partner might actually notice a drastic change in your dopamine levels before you do. But if these symptoms describe how you are feeling right now, it is very likely that you have a dopamine deficiency. This can be caused by genetics, illness, aging, or any of the age accelerators: weight gain, change in memory, stress, or lack of sleep. It doesn't matter what the culprit is, because the fix is the same. The first step to becoming younger and sexier is to enhance your dopamine levels to restore your natural energy. By doing so, your zest for sex will return, and your performance will improve.

I can teach you how to correct a dopamine deficiency just by training your brain to make more dopamine. The more dopamine you have, the more you will want to have sex, and the better you'll be at it. At the same time, with more dopamine your metabolism will run at a steady pace, so that you can stay thin and sexy.

SIGNS OF A LOW DOPAMINE SexQ:

- My performance at work has suffered.
- My genitals seem less sensitive.
- I sometimes experience total exhaustion.
- Sex isn't as satisfying as it used to be.
- I have sex less than once a week.

LOST THE LUST? TEST YOUR SEXUAL FREQUENCY

Sexual frequency is another barometer of your dopamine levels. Choose the answer for each that best describes your thoughts and feelings about sex over the last 8 weeks.

1. **How frequently do you have sexual thoughts?**
   a. Daily
   b. Weekly
   c. Never

2. **Rate your ability to become sexually excited.**
   a. Always able
   b. Sometimes
   c. Unable

3. **How frequently do you initiate sexual activity?**
   a. Very frequently
   b. Sometimes
   c. Never: I wait until I'm asked

4. **Rate your overall degree of sexual satisfaction.**
   a. High
   b. Moderate
   c. Low

5. **How many times in the past 2 months did you engage in:**
   Masturbation:
   a. 2 to 4 times per week or more
   b. 2 to 4 times per month
   c. Less than once a month

   Intercourse:
   a. 2 to 4 times per week or more
   b. 2 to 4 times per month
   c. Less than once a month

   Oral Sex:
   a. 2 to 4 times per week or more
   b. 2 to 4 times per month
   c. Less than once a month

Answers:
If you answered mostly A's, you are high in dopamine; B's reflect a moderate deficiency; C's reflect a major deficiency.

Low Dopamine = High Cortisol = Restless Energy

Have you ever experienced high sexual desire but had difficulty achieving orgasm? A dopamine deficiency may be affecting your cortisol levels. For every brain chemical that becomes deficient, a hormone usually takes its place. The body naturally increases production of the hormone cortisol when there is a dopamine imbalance

Can You Keep Up with the Joneses?

The average couple can engage in sex for 24 minutes. Can you?

Masturbation: Stamina Practice or Narcissistic Wandering?

There are many euphemisms for masturbation, including self-love. I don't oppose masturbation, but I'd rather see you making love with someone else. Still, practice is sometimes necessary. Masturbation can teach you how to recognize the signs of an approaching orgasm. But it isn't a replacement for a deep, loving relationship.

because cortisol is the backup energy hormone: It provides us with additional power so the brain and body can continue to function. Cortisol gets converted to adrenaline and creates the necessary energy the brain and body need.

When cortisol is picking up the slack, you may not realize that you are low on dopamine. You'll continue to feel happy and energetic, but you might also feel restless, because even though cortisol effectively keeps your brain running, it does not improve dopamine levels. All that extra adrenaline can make you feel anxious during the day and unable to sleep at night. Excess cortisol makes you look puffy and round-faced, and it increases your blood pressure and your appetite. It also causes bloating and weight gain, especially in the abdomen. Cortisol is also released when you are under stress, whether or not your dopamine is low. In fact, when you are stressed, you naturally burn more dopamine, causing the release of even more cortisol.

By increasing dopamine, your body will not be forced to rely on cortisol to support its energy needs. Instead, you'll have plenty of sexual energy, desire, and stamina, without the feelings of stress or nervous energy.

What Does a Dopamine Deficiency Feel Like?

Without dopamine you've lost your sexual fire, your metabolic fire, and your intensity to work and play. Low dopamine skin is less sensitive to all types of touch. If you are dopamine deficient, you may find that it takes more time and effort to get things done. Your concentration may wander, your thinking and decision making will not be as quick, and your intensity at work diminishes. Even if you sleep a little longer, you may still wake up tired, needing to reach for a stimulant like coffee just to get yourself going in the morning. The coffee supplies the fix you need to feel like yourself, but the effect is temporary, so you reach for more throughout the day; otherwise you can't sustain your usual level of performance.

Low dopamine sufferers often feel sluggish, even cranky. When we feel this way, we experience an instinctive, often unconscious attempt to bring the fire back. Besides craving caffeine, you may find that you are attracted to foods that will deliver an energy boost: high-sugar, fast-digesting carbohydrates. These actually boost dopamine production, so in one sense you are doing the right thing. Unfortunately, these foods contribute to weight gain, which doesn't make you all that sexy.

Are You Addicted to Sex?

Sex addiction occurs when desire, thoughts, and actions regarding sex negatively affect your everyday life and put your emotional state in jeopardy. Lately, sex addiction has been a hot topic in the media: Tiger Woods, Jesse James, and others have all gone to rehab to fight this very real issue. Like other types of addiction, including those to illegal or prescription drugs, cigarette smoking, drinking, or even aggression, it is a compulsion that is linked to the same underlying disorder: a dopamine brain chemical imbalance.

All of us are vulnerable to the addiction cycle when there is a loss of dopamine. In fact, earlier in my career I worked with Dr. Kenneth Blum, professor of pharmacology at the McNight Brain Institute of the University of Florida College of Medicine; Dr. Ernest P. Noble, the former head of the National Institute on Alcoholism; and Dr. Nora D. Volkow, the current head of the National Institute on Drug Abuse. Our research proved that

Love Releases Dopamine

A 2005 study from Rutgers University scanned the brains of 17 people who were looking at photos of those they loved deeply. The researchers saw an increase in dopamine brain activity similar to that found by addicted cocaine users. This indicates that just recognizing that you are in love boosts dopamine, which boosts your desire.

dopamine genetics predicts a very high predisposition for various addictions. I have also conducted studies that showed that a dysfunction of the D2 dopamine receptors in the brain can lead to addiction, aberrant substance-seeking behaviors, and aggression.

Dopamine works like a natural amphetamine, controlling energy. When you see a person you are strongly attracted to, your dopamine production will naturally spike. And whenever you have sex, your dopamine levels also increase. Both of these scenarios make you feel really good. For those of us with balanced brains, that "dopamine rush" is recognized as satiety or satisfaction.

However, when people who are low in dopamine have sex, they don't feel as satisfied, even if they have an orgasm. Or they interpret the dopamine rush as a euphoric experience that can lead to addiction. The low-dopamine person can be dopamine dependent: She or he needs to have sex more often, or in a variety of ways, or with a variety of people, in order to achieve what others would consider to be a "normal" level of satisfaction. And because they are so turned on by this euphoric sensation, they will seek to replicate the experience over and over again by engaging in more sex. This quest for the dopamine rush creates a sex addiction.

The catch is that the brain can't sustain constant euphoria. Instead, it strives to reach homeostasis, or balance, so that each time we have sex, the brain releases less dopamine. When this happens, the euphoric feeling won't come back at all. Yet low-dopamine people will still continue to have lots of sex, in hope of its returning. In order to break this cycle, low-dopamine people must increase their dopamine in a more balanced approach: first choosing foods, then nutrients, and sometimes even medications, so that sex does not become their only source of happiness.

I often see men in their forties who become sex addicts or highly aggressive individuals when they notice for the first time that their sex life has diminished. When their libido was strong, they were having sex seven or eight times a week. Now, however, they are only having sex once or twice a week, and predict they are on a downward slide. A man might seek out an aggressive encounter in order to experience the rewarding sensation he is missing from sex.

When these men realize they have a problem, they come to see me asking for testosterone, but testosterone alone will not restore brain chemistry. Men who simply take a heavy dose of testosterone don't really learn to manage their health; they are only focusing on getting back to getting more sex. These men are vulnerable to addictions of all types, because their brain has not really been fully balanced. That's why I always pair a prescription of testosterone with what I call the Braverman Protocol: a brain-balanced diet and the nutrients that offset the potency of testosterone.

FOODS THAT DELIVER THE GOODS

The easiest way to dial up your sex life is by eating foods that actually create more dopamine. These foods contain the amino acids, or proteins, that are the building blocks of dopamine. If you are dopamine deficient, you want to focus on foods that are rich in tyrosine and phenylalanine to rev up your dopamine production. Phenylalanine is an essential amino acid found in high-protein foods, such as meats and poultry, dairy products, and wheat germ. The amino acid tyrosine, found in the same

Addicted to Orgasms?

If you are dopamine dependent, you always believe your best orgasm hasn't occurred yet, because you are always looking for the next, better one.

foods, increases your resistance to stress and acts as a natural pain reliever. Most important, tyrosine is an adrenaline builder: Tyrosine can give you the increased energy you may be lacking in bed.

Dopamine-rich foods are also important because when your dopamine is high, so is your metabolism. In order to be younger and sexier, it's quite likely that you need to be thinner as well. My book the *Younger (Thinner) You Diet* provides a comprehensive weight-loss plan based on your brain chemistry. Chapter 12 reviews the basics of that plan so you can begin to lose weight if need be. Remember, being thinner means 15 more years of great sex.

Use the following food list to increase your total phenylalanine and tyrosine intake. You'll need to include protein in each of your three main meals to keep your dopamine high throughout the day.

Phenylalanine can also be found in the sugar substitute aspartame, which is sold under the brand name NutraSweet or Equal. Aspartame has been the subject of more than 200 research studies in the past

Foods That Create Dopamine

FOOD	GRAMS OF DOPAMINE PRECURSORS PER 6–8 OZ SERVING
Wild game	4.10
Cottage cheese	3.40
Pork	2.50
Wheat germ	2.35
Turkey	2.30
Duck	2.20
Chicken	2.00
Ricotta cheese	1.85
Walnuts	1.40
Soy products	1.20
Beef, lean	1.10
Granola	1.05
Oatmeal	0.85
Chocolate, dark	0.80
Yogurt	0.80
Eggs (1 egg)	0.60

Eggs Are a Symbol of Fertility for a Reason

Both bird and fish eggs are high in phenylalanine and tyrosine, as well as B vitamins, which help to balance hormones and fight stress. They are also high in protein to give you more energy in bed.

30 years, and its safety continues to be demonstrated.

Spice Up Your Sex Life

Spices are nutrient dense: Each one can provide between 20 and 80 different nutrients. By eating some at every meal, you are benefiting by adding important vitamins, minerals, and even antioxidants to your diet. They allow your foods to be metabolized better because calories are burned more easily when they are accompanied by nutrients.

I love to mix a variety of spices in each meal, and I often tell my patients about Trader Joe's 21 Spice Salute, which, as you could guess, contains 21 different spices. Total Health Nutrients (www.totalhealth nutrients.com) also offers dozens of spice combinations. You'll learn more about the power of spices in Chapter 12, but the bottom line is that fresh spices are one of the greatest defenses against aging.

What's more, certain spices are known to heat up your sex drive. For example, chile peppers contain capsaicin, known to stimulate nerve endings. They are also thought to release endorphins, giving you

that "runner's high." Garlic contains allicin, which increases blood flow to your genitals.

The following can boost your dopamine level and spice up your sex life.

- Basil
- Black pepper
- Cayenne
- Chile peppers
- Cumin
- Fennel
- Flaxseeds
- Garlic
- Ginger
- Mustard seed
- Rosemary
- Savory
- Sesame seeds
- Tarragon
- Turmeric

Boost Your Sexual Stamina with Caffeine

Coffee definitely boosts your dopamine as well as your sex drive, because it gets your blood pumping. It also enhances endurance by releasing fat stored in the body so you can have sex for longer periods of time. But for the healthiest caffeine option, I prefer tea to coffee.

Teas are healthier than sodas or coffee because they are also high in nutrients and antioxidants, yet they don't contain a single calorie. Tea also contains L-theanine, which actually helps to relax you. In order to have great sex, you need to achieve the perfect combination of stimulation and relaxation in order to let go completely and truly enjoy yourself.

Choose your teas wisely. Tea freshly brewed from loose tea leaves has far more nutrients than tea made from tea bags. Bottled tea beverages may also be diluted or sweetened, adding unnecessary calories. My book the *Younger (Thinner) You Diet* includes everything you need to know about teas and their various properties.

NEW SUPPLEMENTS THAT WILL DRIVE YOU WILD

Readily available vitamins and nutrient supplements are an excellent way to ensure a steady supply of dopamine. Because the supplements that boost dopamine are energy-related, they are best taken on a full stomach after you've eaten breakfast or lunch.

Phenylalanine and tyrosine are also available as supplements but by themselves offer weak dopamine replenishment. However, when combined in a formula with the herb rhodiola, they can create a very efficient sex enhancer.

Everyone's Talking about Maca

Maca is a radishlike plant that has shown to be a tremendous libido enhancer. It possesses specific chemical compounds that support enhanced sexual function. Maca had been used in Peru for generations to enhance fertility and increase energy and libido. It also helps to increase stamina and endurance. It works to balance hormone levels in the body by supporting the pituitary gland, which in turn, helps the body produce more hormones. As a result, estrogen, progesterone, and testosterone levels are raised.

The herb was considered so potent that the Incas reserved its use for their royal family. Today, the Scottish publication *Herbal News* calls this natural aphrodisiac "the female Viagra," and a double-blind 2008 study at Massachusetts General Hospital concluded that it has a "beneficial effect on libido."

Maca is available as a supplement on its own, or as an ingredient in a combination supplement like Super Miraforte, which I often recommend to my patients. This new supplement contains high potencies of maca as well as chrysin and nettle root—plant extracts that naturally reduce the conversion of testosterone to estrogen, which will then enhance testosterone levels. It also contains muira puama, another rain forest herb classified as an aphrodisiac. In a trial of men with decreased libido and other sexual

Double Dopamine Power

Try steeping two green tea bags in 2 cups of boiling water and adding a pinch of cayenne. Put the tea in a thermos and you can drink it all day long.

issues, 62 percent of those taking muira puama reported positive results in regard to libido, while 51 percent of those with a common sexual problem felt that the herb was helpful. A second trial examined men with decreased libido and found that 85 percent of the test subjects taking muira puama enjoyed an enhanced libido, 90 percent had improved sexual function, and 100 percent of test subjects experienced an increase in intercourse frequency. Maca is also available commercially in several forms, including powder, liquid, tablets, and capsules. The recommended dose is one 450 milligram capsule of dried maca extract three times daily, taken orally with food. Do not take this supplement if you have prostate cancer.

Dopamine-Boosting Sex Enhancers

I'm sure you've seen all kinds of advertisements for "pill form" sexual enhancers, either on television or in magazines. Most of them don't work. Look at their ingredients carefully, and see if they contain any of the following. These supplements have been known to enhance desire and libido. While you don't need a doctor's prescription to buy these, you do need to know how they will affect your health, especially if you have already been diagnosed with chronic illness or disease. Discuss all of these options with your doctor and choose together which ones may be best for you. Read carefully to see if they will improve your current health status as well as your sexual function.

NATURAL TREATMENTS	SUGGESTED DAILY DOSAGE	HOW IT AFFECTS SEX
Arginine	1,000–20,000 mg	Can help men increase the frequency and lasting time of erections. Choose if you have vascular problems to increase blood flow.
Boron	1–5 mg	Increases sexual desire in women, amplifying intensity of orgasm. Will also help if you have osteoporosis and if you are losing height.
Folic acid	500 mcg	Increases dopamine levels in the brain, enhancing libido. A good choice for women on birth control or people with depression, alcohol issues, or anxiety.

NATURAL TREATMENTS	SUGGESTED DAILY DOSAGE	HOW IT AFFECTS SEX
Ginkgo biloba	100–200 mg	Ginkgo's three major pharmacological features all enhance libido: improving the blood supply to the brain, reducing the potential for blood clotting, and increasing dopamine production. Recommended for those with circulation problems.
Ginseng	500–2,000 mg	This Asian root has been proven to enhance sexual performance and improve libido by facilitating blood flow to the penis and the brain. It also improves adrenal malfunction, DHEA deficiency, and autoimmune diseases.
Guarana	200–1,000 mg	Contains a natural form of caffeine that is 2.5 times stronger than coffee and tea. This supplement stimulates the adrenal gland to release dopamine into the blood stream. Helps to resolve fatigue and depression.
L-Dopa	200–500 mg	Precursor to dopamine. Used for patients with Parkinson's, chronic fatigue, or memory loss.
Maca	1,000–3,000 mg	Improves ejaculate or low sex drive.
Methionine	500–2,000 mg	Elevates mood, which may increase desire for sex. Can be used to reverse depression, fatigue, fatty liver, and arthritis.
Phenylalanine	500–4,000 mg	Precursor to dopamine. Used to reverse pain.
Phosphatidylserine	200–400 mg	Can increase dopamine levels, lower cortisol, and aid memory loss.
Rhodiola rosea	50–750 mg	Promotes physical and mental energy. Can be used for depression, fatigue, and attention deficit disorder (ADD).
Thiamin (vitamin B$_1$)	100–500 mg	Increases dopamine levels in the brain, enhancing libido.

(continued)

(continued)

NATURAL TREATMENTS	SUGGESTED DAILY DOSAGE	HOW IT AFFECTS SEX
Tyrosine	500–4,000 mg	Precursor to dopamine. Addresses fatigue, depression, and ADD.
Yohimbe	200–400 mg	Facilitates erections by stimulating the nervous system and increasing blood flow to the penis. Contains dopamine-related compounds and is effective for treating male impotence. It can also reduce emotional issues.
Zinc	30–120 mg	Increases sexual desire in men, increasing intensity of orgasm. Should be taken if you are living in an urban area with high amounts of toxic metals.

DIAL UP YOUR SEX LIFE WITH NATURAL BIOIDENTICAL HORMONES

Most doctors will look to medicine to "cure" a problem. However, drugs that have been proven to alter dopamine levels are highly addictive and therefore not the preferred method of treating this deficiency. For most men and women, natural hormone supplementation is the key to enhancing dopamine as well as desire.

Hormone supplements work as nutrients that feed your aging brain, because as you age, your own production of hormones slowly diminishes. Replacing lost hormones not only rejuvenates the body, but they actually enhance the production of specific brain chemicals, including dopamine.

The trend in recent years is toward natural bioidentical hormone compounds, often from plant sources, as opposed to synthetic compounds. The molecular structures of bioidentical hormones are identical to those of the actual hormones produced by the human body. Bioidentical therapies are generally very safe, bearing little health risk, unlike their synthetic counterparts, and are so lacking in side effects that many are sold as over-the-counter supplements.

The most exciting hormone therapies for enhancing desire and improving stamina are those that are directly related to dopamine: testosterone, leptin, DHEA, and human growth hormone (HGH). Ellie Capria and my team at PATH Medical have helped me create hormone-enhancing programs for both men and women that help them regain their youthful sexual vibrancy.

TESTOSTERONE PUMPS YOU UP

Testosterone is a sex hormone produced by the adrenal glands as well as the ovaries and testes. Testosterone levels increase naturally with regular sexual activity. However, like all hormones, its production begins to wane with age. The testosterone level of a 20-year-old woman is approximately twice as high as that of a 40-year-old. Other factors, including birth control pills, can also lower testosterone levels. For men, the production of testosterone begins around the time of puberty and slowly decreases in their thirties, dropping about 1 percent every year after that.

A high dopamine SexQ is likely to have high testosterone levels. For example, I recently treated a 44-year-old woman who had only 9 percent body fat—less than I had ever seen before. Even more surprising, she had the sex drive of a 22-year-old. She wanted to have sex at least once a day. When I tested her blood, it showed that her testosterone level was seven times higher than that of a typical woman her age.

Testosterone is directly linked to dopamine, and therefore it is connected to sexual desire and performance. If you had a high dopamine SexQ and now notice that your sexual desire is lagging, you might be losing your testosterone and aging prematurely. The good news is that both men and women can increase their testosterone levels safely and experience an increase in sexual desire and ability. I also prescribe it to men and women to increase their assertiveness and confidence. What's more, testosterone therapies also improve your overall health, helping to combat extreme tiredness, low energy, depression, and brittle bones. Testosterone is also used in weight management, as it facilitates weight loss by inhibiting body-fat storage, especially in the abdomen.

Synthetically produced testosterone was first introduced as methyl testosterone, but it was pulled from the market long ago because of its link to liver cancer. Instead, natural testosterone produced from plant sources is safe and widely available through a prescription. I have found that the best results for women as well as men are gained through the testosterone patch or testosterone cream.

Men apply testosterone creams and gels to their shoulders and arms, or lower

Soak Up Some Sun

Just 20 minutes of real spring/summer sunlight (or year-round if you live in warmer climates) per day without sunscreen causes the production of the skin pigment melanin (made from tyrosine), which can heat up your libido and lend a bit of staying power. Dr. James Watson at the University of California found that male patients injected with melanin "developed sustained and unprovoked erections."

stomach. Women use minute amounts of topical cream directly on the clitoris. This application can enlarge the clitoris because it improves blood flow and stretches nerve endings, which enhances sensitivity and heightens the physical sensations of sex. Women quickly find that their ability to become sexually aroused increases significantly.

The Downsides of Testosterone

It is important to have your blood levels monitored by your doctor when using testosterone. Overmedication can cause blood clots, pulmonary embolisms, deep vein thrombosis, rage, and mood swings in both men and women. I've seen women overuse testosterone and then grow facial hair, or have their judgment clouded by an overwhelming need for sex.

Another negative side effect of testosterone is that both men and women can become addicted to it, with devastating results. I once met a famous surgeon at a conference whose physique was incredible: He had turned himself into a muscle-bound monster at the age of 65. I asked him what he was taking, and he told me that he was "loading up on testosterone." But the downside was severe: His testosterone addiction made him addicted to sex. He was delighted to tell me all about his most recent sexual escapades. At the time, he was flying to the Philippines to have sex with 14-year-old girls. Eventually, the testoster-

one thickened his blood and he died of an aneurysm.

Here's another example. A 58-year-old man came to see an antiaging doctor whom I had trained, complaining of low sex drive. The young doctor put this man on a high dose of testosterone cream. The man's wife soon felt her own sex drive could not keep up with her husband's improved vigor and desire for sex. After seeing his results, she started using his medication, even though this dose was much too high for a woman of her size and age. To her delight she noticed very quickly that her sex life improved: Her vaginal muscles enlarged, her clitoris enlarged, and she was able to enjoy sex with her husband and match his libido with renewed desire of her own.

Unfortunately, unmonitored testosterone use can increase risk-taking behaviors. The couple became addicted to sex. They started taking prostitutes into their bed, traveling to Thailand on sex vacations, and engaging in dangerous behaviors.

The negative side effects of testosterone can be avoided under the right supervision if the treating physician understands that only a balanced brain leads to balanced sex. If these people had been given testosterone along with serotonin agents to offset some of the effects of the testosterone, they wouldn't have needed testosterone at such high dosages to get the renewed sexual vigor they were after. If doctors had investigated their acetylcholine and other

Typical Testosterone Dosages

For Men Bioidentical varieties only: • Compounded Gel • AndroGel • Injectable	5%, 10%, 15%, 20%, up to 1 to 2 squirts a day
For Women Choose bioidentical varieties only: • Topical cream	0.5% to 1%, 2.5–10 mg daily (apply a lentil-size amount to the clitoris 30 minutes prior to intercourse)

important cognitive markers, they would have been able to prescribe a treatment that would have worked without pushing them into dangerous territory.

LEPTIN MAKES YOU THIN AND SEXY

Any amount of extra weight that you are currently carrying will adversely affect your sex life. But while it's true that being overweight can make you too tired to have sex, and you may be uninterested or disinclined because you're self-conscious about your body, there may be a biological cause that links excess weight to lack of libido, and that's the hormone leptin. As leptin levels rise, changes occur throughout the brain, reducing the effectiveness of dopamine and, in response, dampening your sex drive and your sexual response.

Leptin is secreted by your own fat tissue. Its job is to communicate with the brain about your energy stores by sending signals when you have reached satiety, or fullness, so that you stop eating. After leptin is released, your brain receives the message through specific leptin receptors. Then, when the brain gets the message, you are supposed to stop eating. The level of leptin in your body is dependent upon whether your fat cells are secreting it appropriately, and if your leptin receptors are receiving the right message. However, if you are obese, or overeat regularly, your leptin receptors may not be sensitive to the leptin message, and your brain won't tell your body to stop eating. This is referred to as leptin resistance, which in turn leads to a dopamine response that impedes weight loss because it increases hunger and food-seeking behavior. These behaviors can lead to further accumulation of body fat, which is then linked to an increased risk of heart disease, diabetes, and other conditions (and their related medications) that also contribute to the destruction of your sex life.

You can find out if you have leptin resistance with a simple blood test. Low leptin levels are ideal: It is an indicator that you may actually be carrying less body fat than your body mass index (BMI) presents, because you have more muscle than body fat.

Low leptin people will generally have higher dopamine levels and good sexual energy. When dopamine and even testosterone levels increase, leptin levels decrease, increasing libido for both sexes. It may turn out to be true that the thin have more sex, because they have less leptin.

However, when leptin levels are high, you will continue to accumulate more body fat. When this happens, you become both leptin resistant *and* sexually resistant. When leptin levels increase, serotonin increases, which makes you less driven to have sex. For women, this manifests as a general loss of sexual interest. For men, it increases the time it takes for ejaculation.

Another reason it's important to know your leptin level is that it can be used as an indicator of overall health. A 2010 study I was involved with was the first large-scale comparison between BMI and DEXA, a direct measure of percentage body fat. BMI is based solely on height and weight and may misclassify individuals if they have disproportionately high or low amounts of body fat. DEXA scans, on the other hand, can measure fat exactly, in every part of the body. DEXA scans are particularly effective for men and women who are "thin but unfit," a condition known as normal-weight obesity, in which BMI is low but there is actually a high percentage of body fat present in comparison to muscle. These individuals are also at risk for an impaired sex life, because even though they look thin, their lack of muscle tone (particularly for women) means they are carrying extra and unnecessary body fat, and possibly higher leptin levels.

The Centers for Disease Control and Prevention (CDC) traditionally considers adults with a BMI between 25 and 29.9 overweight, while adults with a BMI of 30 or higher are obese. In this study, DEXA scans were able to accurately measure that 56 percent of the participants in the study were obese, while BMI indentified only 20 percent. Furthermore, 5 percent of the participants who were initially identified as obese by BMI measurement were reclassified as non-obese. Direct fat measurements from DEXA are clearly superior and have the additional benefit of showing body fat distribution, which is particularly important because percentage of body fat and its distribution is the best predictor of longevity.

DEXA scans are extremely accurate, but they are also expensive and time-consuming, and therefore not widely available to all patients. We found that monitoring leptin levels in conjunction with the BMI greatly improved the accuracy measuring obesity, at a fraction of the cost of a DEXA scan. Hopefully, in the not too distant future, knowing your leptin score will become a common part of your annual physical. Obesity is a medical disease, and we can use leptin measurement as a tool to diagnose it. It is just as important as knowing your blood sugar levels or hemoglobin A1C if you are monitoring diabetes, or blood pressure for controlling hypertension.

Potential Factors That Raise Leptin Levels and Lower Your Libido

HEALTH CONCERNS	ELEVATED TRIGLYCERIDE LEVELS
Drugs	• Cocaine and amphetamines
	• Decadron (dexamethasone)
	• Depakote (valproate)
	• DiaBeta (glibenclamide)
	• Hydrocortisone
	• Neurontin (gabapentin)
	• Risperdal (risperidone)
	• Seroquel (quetiapine)
	• Tenormin (atenolol)
Lifestyle	• Decreased sleep
	• Increased stress

Factors That Can Help Lower Leptin Levels

	AGENT
Nutritional Supplements	• Acetyl-l-carnitine
	• Carnitine (easily found as a powder)
	• Conjugated linoleic acid
	• Integra-Lean (irvingia)
	• Melatonin
	• Omega-3 fatty acids
	• Resveratrol
	• Vitamin D
Dietary Changes	• A 12-week low-glycemic-index diet
	• 1 mM eicosapentaenoic acid or DHA
	• Increased consumption of fish
	• Increased consumption of vegetables
	• Increased intake of dietary fiber
	• Lower caloric intake
	• N-3 polyunsaturated fatty acids
	• Removing dietary fructose

(continued)

(continued)

	AGENT
Lifestyle Changes	• At least 7 hours of sleep each night • Decreasing stress • Increasing physical activity
Pharmaceutical Choices	• Altace (ramipril) • Atacand (Candesartan) • Avandia (rosiglitazone) • Byetta (exenatide) • D2 leptin stabilizer • Detantol (bunazosin hydrochloride) • Diovan (valsartan) • Dopaminergic agents • Glucophage (metformin) • Landel (efonidipine) • Lipitor (atorvastatin) • Metopirone (metyrapone) • Metreleptin (leptin analog) • Norvasc (amlodipine) • Omacor (omega-3 polyunsaturated fatty acids) • Parlodel (bromocriptine) • Retin-A (all-trans retinoic acid) • Symlin (amylin analog) • Victoza (liraglutide) • Visken (pindolol)
Hormone Balancing	• Increased DHEA • Increased testosterone • Lower estrogen

Better still, we are now able to change your leptin levels by following the Braverman Protocol. Talk with your doctor about the information in the previous chart in order to pair the best treatment options that match your current health so that you can become thinner and sexier.

Increase Testosterone Naturally with Easy Lifestyle Changes

The most natural way to increase testosterone levels is through diet and regular exercise, and it's never too early to start. Since your testosterone declines at a steady rate, it's more than likely that boosting your hormone levels naturally, even in your twenties and thirties, could help you maintain higher levels later on.

Get rid of the belly: Carrying excess body fat elevates estrogen levels, which may cause your testosterone to sink. However, slow and steady weight loss is the way to go. Your body still needs real calories to make testosterone, so regularly skipping meals or going for long stretches without eating can cause your hormone levels to plummet. Your goal should be to lose no more than 1 pound a week.

Try tough exercise for lots of love: Testosterone levels will increase when your workout includes plenty of strength training. Focus on "compound" weight-lifting exercises that train several large muscle groups. Studies have shown that doing squats, bench presses, or back rows increases testosterone more than doing biceps curls or triceps pushdowns, even though the effort may seem the same.

Discuss any weight-bearing exercise program with your doctor before you begin. If you get the go-ahead, start by using a heavy weight that you can lift only five times. That weight is about 85 percent of your one-repetition maximum. A Finnish study found that this workload produced the greatest boosts in testosterone. Then, do three sets of each weight-lifting movement, as researchers at Penn State have determined that this fosters greater increases in testosterone than just one or two sets. Rest a full minute between sets, so you can regain strength to continue lifting at least 70 percent of your one-rep maximum during the second and third sets.

Rest harder than you work out: If you don't allow your body to recuperate adequately between training sessions, your circulating testosterone levels can plunge by as much as 40 percent, according to a study at the University of North Carolina. The symptoms of overtraining are hard to miss: irritability, insomnia, and muscle shrinkage. To avoid overtraining, make sure you sleep a full 8 hours at night, and never stress the same muscles with weight-lifting movements 2 days in a row.

Stay off the sauce: In order to maintain a healthy testosterone level, cut yourself off after three drinks. Alcohol can kill testosterone levels because it affects the endocrine system.

DHEA: TESTOSTERONE'S BFF

The hormone DHEA normally spikes right before orgasm to enhance desire and focus, and it may increase dopamine production. Produced by the adrenal glands, testicles, and brain, DHEA (dehydroepiandrosterone) is the precursor to all sex hormones, which is why it plays an important role for both men and women. Many people complain that when they have intercourse, they're tired, or they are too tired to even engage in sex. The hormones of the adrenal gland are important for reversing that fatigue, giving you more energy to have better sex.

DHEA levels peak in your twenties and thirties and then begin to decline. By the time you reach 70, these levels are down by 20 percent. Determination of DHEA levels is sometimes a more accurate indicator of sexual dysfunction than testosterone testing. Reestablishing DHEA gives people wilder, more energetic sex. DHEA controls a woman's sex drive more than any other hormone, as it converts to estrogen and testosterone. For men, DHEA acts as a mild androgen, also promoting sexual activity. Its influence on sexual function is similar to testosterone.

Recent studies have shown that both men and women can enjoy the enhanced sexual benefits of DHEA treatment aimed at restoring the original youthful levels. When DHEA is used in conjunction with testosterone therapy, it enhances the benefits of testosterone and reduces the negative side effects. Two weeks of DHEA replacement in healthy men and women resulted in DHEA levels returning to those of young adulthood: Sexually, noticeable changes were evident in both desire and performance. Taking a DHEA supplement an hour before sex significantly increased both mental and physical arousal in postmenopausal women, according to a study published in the *Journal of Women's Health and Gender-Based Medicine*.

GROWTH HORMONE KEEPS YOUR SEX LIFE STRONG

HGH is produced by the pituitary gland. Growth hormone does not have growth properties and instead functions throughout the body as a repair hormone. It increases all aspects of brain electrical function, from brain speed and processing to the creation of the sex hormones. It lends a hand in forming new muscle cells, new blood components, and better metabolism, giving you a tremendous sexual advantage by repairing the entire brain and body, and keeping your other sex hormones high. Growth hormone supplementation has been associated with increased libido, pleasure in response, and potential for multiple orgasms.

Growth hormone is also critical for tissue repair, muscle growth, brain function, immune system function, physical and mental health, and bone strength. It has been shown to affect the brain's abilities in cognition, emotion, and mood, and boost cellular metabolism, leading to increased energy, which has a decisive impact upon increasing sexual interest and ability.

Case Study: Carl and Gail Found Sex More Fun at 60

Gail and Carl first came to see me 2 years ago, when Gail was 56 and Carl was 61. A doctor himself who was interested in anti-aging medicine, Carl had read about my work in *Life Extension* magazine, and they came all the way from western New York State to see me. The office visit was Carl's birthday gift to Gail. Carl had begun to notice that Gail wasn't acting quite like her old self. And the fact of the matter was, neither was he.

Gail came into my office with very troubling news. She had been diagnosed with severe osteoporosis, which concerned her because she and Carl were very athletic, and her doctor had told her that she would have to give up skiing. Gail's parents were still alive at ages 90 and 94; Carl's mother lived until she was 97. Gail knew that longevity was on their side, but she was beginning to regard the future with concern and trepidation. She didn't want to live 30 or 40 years longer if she couldn't stay active. Gail told me that she hadn't been sleeping well for a long time, and that she had recently gained weight. Even though she believed that she was past menopause, her local physician had recommended that she take synthetic estrogen, but Gail was wary. She had also tried several over-the-counter remedies for osteoporosis, including calcium, strontium, boron, and vitamin D, but nothing helped. At the end of the initial interview, Gail also confided in me that her sex life was suffering. She told me that the couple used to enjoy an active sex life, but now they were both avoiding sex and only getting together once a week or every other week. In fact, Gail, who had been the one with a stronger libido, was happy that her husband had little interest in sex, because sex for her had become so physically uncomfortable.

The minute I understood her full patient history I knew that I needed to treat both Carl and Gail. I called Carl into the office and did a full checkup on him as well. Carl's testosterone levels were very low, which is why his sex life was destroyed. I then explained to this couple that their SexQ had changed completely as they had aged. They were thrilled to hear that by following my protocol, they would both be able to reverse the aging that had occurred to Gail's bones and hormonal levels and to Carl's declining testosterone.

I started Gail on a natural hormone replacement, including a topical testosterone cream, an estrogen patch, and oral progesterone. I prescribed Forteo to strengthen her bones and growth hormone to increase muscle mass. I also noticed that she had low thyroid levels and treated that as well.

Initially, I put Carl on a very low dose of topical testosterone because I wanted to match their SexQ: I guessed that Gail wouldn't respond to her treatment as quickly as Carl, and I didn't think that she was ready for him to have a full sex drive. A month later, Gail called and asked if I could increase Carl's testosterone dosage: Carl wasn't able to keep up with her sexual needs. I obliged happily.

Within a few months Gail reported to me that she was sleeping better. She had lost 15 pounds without dieting as her muscle mass increased and her body fat decreased. And she was beaming when she told me about the changes she was noticing in their sex life. By following the hormone regimen, both Carl and Gail felt that their sex life had become as active as it was in the earliest years of their marriage. They were enjoying each other immensely, having sex every day, sometimes twice a day.

Two years later, Gail still believes that their first office visit was the best birthday present Carl has ever given her. Her bone density has improved tremendously, and she's been able to stop taking Forteo. Each told me they feel like young kids again. Carl is retiring soon, and Gail is thrilled at the thought of having him home all the time. Her energy is back, and she's never felt better. Physically she feels 10 to 20 years younger.

I gradually increased Carl's testosterone dosage to a stable level. Carl feels that he has the energy now to keep up with his busy schedule and to keep up with Gail. The last time I saw them, they were planning a big ski trip with their three grown boys, and Gail and Carl were looking forward to seeing if they could keep up with them on the slopes.

DOPAMINE MEDICATIONS CAN RESTORE YOUR SEX LIFE

Traditional medications can help return the brain's chemistry to a more normal level. Some work because they imitate a particular brain chemical, triggering the brain to respond as if it were producing dopamine itself. Others block the brain chemical from being absorbed, making the brain chemical more available to the brain and the body.

Amphetamines like Adderall and Ritalin improve sexuality. Wellbutrin, a dopamine reuptake inhibitor, works, as do a number of prescription drugs that may act as sex stimulants. In a 1996 German study, a number of drugs were discussed for their potential aphrodisiac properties, including levodopa (L-dopa), amantadine, pergolide, naloxone, naltrexone, and imipramine. Clomiphene (Clomid) and tamoxifen (Nolvadex) are both antiestrogenics that cause the secretion of growth hormone as well as increase testosterone concentration, thereby increasing libido.

The following medications are currently prescribed to work with dopamine to increase sexual desire and stamina. Discuss them with your doctor to determine if they are necessary, and if they will affect other health issues you may be experiencing.

- **Adderall, Ritalin, Concerta, and Dexedrine** are amphetamines that are also prescribed for depression, ADD, and fatigue.
- **Amantadine** is an antiviral medication, also prescribed for Parkinson's disease.
- **Apomorphine** is considered an experimental medication. It may enhance sexual performance for both men and women, including enhancing erections, by selectively activating dopamine receptors.
- **Bupropion** (Wellbutrin) is a powerful antidepressant that increases sexual desire for men and women by enhancing the availability of dopamine and working as its preservative. A study reported in 2009 in the *Journal of Sex and Marital Therapy* found that nearly one-third of participants who took bupropion reported more desire, arousal, and fantasy.
- **Deprenyl and Eldepryl** may increase male and female sexual desire by enhancing dopamine. It is commonly used to treat depression, Parkinson's disease, and dementia.
- **Flibanserin** was originally marketed as an antidepressant but was found by researchers at the University of North Carolina to increase libido in rats as well as humans. It is currently being investigated as a potential treatment for hypoactive sexual desire disorder (HSDD) in premenopausal women, although it has not achieved FDA approval.
- **Naloxone** is also prescribed to combat drug opioid addiction.
- **Naltrexone** is also prescribed to treat narcotic drug and alcohol addiction.
- **Nolvadex, Istubal, and Valodex** (tamoxifen) are also used to treat early breast cancer.
- **Norpramin, Effexor, and Cymbalta** are antidepressant and antianxiety medications.
- **Pergolide and Levodopa** (L–dopa) are also prescribed for Parkinson's disease.
- **Provigil** also treats fatigue and sleepiness.
- **Strattera** is also used for treating attention-deficit hyperactivity disorder (ADHD).
- **Tofranil** (imipramine) is a tricyclic antidepressant that can increase sexual desire.

NICOTINE PUTS AN END TO A GREAT SexQ

Nicotine initially helps to get your sex drive up, as it increases dopamine and leptin. But in the long run it destroys acetylcholine and your ability to become aroused. If for no other reason than that (and there are plenty), you must quit smoking now. Just don't replace one bad habit with another; you can't justify eating or drinking more because you're trying to quit smoking.

Instead, get professional help. There are great medications out there, like varenicline (Chantix) that your doctor can prescribe to help end your addiction to cigarettes once and for all. Also, many of the treatments I describe here that will increase your sex drive, including Wellbutrin, Effexor, and testosterone, will also lessen your appetite for nicotine.

DIAL DOWN YOUR SexQ

Believe it or not, there will be times when having a high dopamine SexQ is less than ideal. For example, your partner might not be ready yet for your increased libido, or he or she might prefer a gentler, more intimate type of sexual relationship. You might have adult ADD, which leads to a "wandering eye" that can't focus sexually on just one partner, or you put off having sex even though you want it. If you have been told that you are overly dominant in bed, decreasing your dopamine levels helps you take a different role. And if a crisis such as a serious illness prevents you from having sex with your partner, you may need to tone things down before you find yourself on the couch. If your dopamine levels are truly sky-high, you can have a spontaneous orgasm without sexual provocation, which is messy, to say the least.

You know you need to turn your sex style down if it's either interfering with your relationship or it's interfering with your life. Too much dopamine allows the libido to go wild. If your whole life revolves around sex, and you are focused on trying to have orgasms all day long, you'll end up stressed and anxious, which is exactly what sex is supposed to counteract.

The good news is that it's just as easy to dial back your brain chemistry as it is to augment it. You can become the lover that is just right for your partner. All you need to do is decrease your dopamine and increase your acetylcholine, GABA, and serotonin.

More acetylcholine makes you feel more romantic and improves your emotional IQ so you can be more present, more engaged, more connected with your spouse. More GABA allows you to relax, become steadier, less demanding. More serotonin allows you to become more playful, take yourself less seriously, and have more fun in bed. While sex ultimately increases all of your brain chemistry, following the lessons in Chapters 5, 6, and 7 will get these specific brain chemicals up so you can have relational, meaningful sex, instead of empty sex.

To lower a SexQ, I often prescribe supplements like St. John's wort, tryptophan, and inositol to lower libido. There are even medications that suppress sexuality by blocking dopamine, including:

- Aldactone

- Antiandrogens (like medroxyprogesterone)

- Antidepressant SSRIs such as Paxil, Zoloft, Celexa, Prozac, Luvox, Lexapro

- Antipsychotics

- Avodart

- Clomipramine

- Clonidine

- Propecia

Now that you understand what a dopamine imbalance looks and feels like, you can start to follow the program. Give yourself a few weeks to see if you—or your partner—notice significant changes. When you enhance your dopamine, you'll almost immediately feel that you have more internal power. Your sex life will change too. You'll have more energy for sex and a greater capacity to have sex more often. Hopefully this will lead to positive changes within your relationship, returning you and your partner to a more intimate lifestyle.

CHAPTER 5

Acetylcholine Enhances Your Technique

YOUR BRAIN'S SPEED—how quickly electrical signals from the brain to the body are processed—is governed by the brain-chemical family hallmarked by acetylcholine. It directly affects how fast we think and how we retain information. While acetylcholine is not as powerful as dopamine in terms of regulating sexual desire, it is related to arousal, the "let's get going" feeling you have when you want to have sex.

When acetylcholine levels are optimal, brain speed is high and you'll have superior cognitive functioning, especially with your memory and attention. You will be abundantly creative and connect romantically with your partner or spouse. Just thinking about your partner will turn you on. High levels of acetylcholine give you the active imagination necessary to keep you excited and interested in your marriage, because without creativity, how can the 2,600th intimate event between any couple still be exciting? The reason is simple: Sex is all about technique and imagination.

The acetylcholine SexQ is defined by adventure. It can lead men who fantasize about becoming explorers to bring that mind-set into the bedroom, where they notch the bedposts with new conquests. These same men, however, can become bored with sex when they are in long-term relationships. For women, the acetylcholine SexQ can become a trap, causing sex to happen only when everything is "just perfect": They need romance, candles, the right wine, the sexy outfit, and an intense, loving bond to get in the mood.

As we all know, such a scenario isn't always attainable. That shouldn't mean that we stop having sex with the same partner, or that we have to wait for the perfect moment. Instead we have to broaden our capacity to create situations conducive to great sex. Creativity doesn't have to mean someone or something new; it can simply mean changing your expectations.

An acetylcholine deficiency occurs when your brain is either burning too

Acetylcholine Sexual Archetypes

Too high: Greta Garbo—low dopamine, but high acetylcholine romantic idealism: She just wanted to be left alone.
Too low: Clara Barton—in combination with high GABA: She was the founder of the Red Cross and spent her energy taking care of everyone but neglected her own love life.

much acetylcholine or not producing enough. Both dopamine and acetylcholine act as electrical "on" switches for the brain: They create energy the body uses for power and speed. When your brain speed slows, you react less quickly to sensory stimuli. This causes forgetfulness, as your brain can't connect new stimuli to previously stored memories or thoughts. Some people describe this as "brain fog." Memory and attention disturbances can cause us to make bad choices, especially when starting new relationships.

People with acetylcholine deficiencies may also find themselves unable to concentrate and focus on the enjoyment of sex, which affects your ability to become aroused. Stimulation and arousal suffer because you have a hard time connecting emotionally. Your body's sexual signals take too long to get you going, or they fizzle out before you can have a meaningful experience. You might also feel less creative in all aspects of life and stop viewing yourself as a sexual person.

Low levels of acetylcholine may result in the body's inability to produce enough internal lubrication; we literally dry out, or in the case of sex, dry up. This affects vaginal lubrication in women, which in turn leads to painful intercourse and a lowered

desire for sex. That's why many women like to apply massage oil before making love, because they equate that slippery lubrication oil with high romance. Lower moisture levels can also adversely affect semen volume in men.

Of all the brain chemicals, a loss of acetylcholine is one of the easiest to spot. And you won't have to wait for your spouse or partner to let you know that something is wrong: You'll notice that you're not feeling like yourself. You may be finding that what was once a romantic turn-on at 22 no longer does it for you. Once upon a time, if you went on a fantastic date, you were ready for sex when you got home. Today, your attitude might be closer to "you want me to do what for a bunch of flowers?" It's not that you don't love your spouse: The arousal bar is just higher because your brain chemistry has changed.

By ramping up your acetylcholine levels, you can boost your brain speed as well as your internal lubrication, allowing sex once again to be smooth, gliding, and thoughtful. You'll feel more alert and will think faster, and your sexual creativity and romantic nature will return. You may also experience an improvement to your memory, attention, and IQ, and your brain fog will naturally dissipate. All of this will help you feel younger, smarter, and sexier.

SIGNS OF A LOW ACETYLCHOLINE SexQ:

- I'm not turned on by touch or massage.
- I misinterpret people's emotions.
- My skin is dry and cracked.
- Sometimes I don't remember what I've eaten.
- I've only had a handful of sexual partners.

AROUSAL SHOULD COME EASILY AT ANY AGE

Your brain's electricity connects your body's physical experiences to memories and thoughts. In a sense, that is the definition of sexual arousal. Arousal is the period between desire and climax, where the brain and body get ready for sex. It is triggered by both psychological and physical stimuli: the thoughts you have about an upcoming sexual act as well as your response to touch, smell, taste, sound, and sight. The ability to achieve arousal requires a creative, fast-thinking brain so that you can quickly remember what turns you on, and then respond accordingly.

Each of these physical responses is connected to acetylcholine, which helps to create the internal lubrication that allows for better blood flow throughout the brain (for better thinking) and the body. And, it supplies the external lubrication you need to make sex comfortable and skin touchably soft. For men, the added moisture of

You know you're aroused when you experience the following:

For men	For women
• Erect nipples	• Erect nipples
• Erect penis	• Firm clitoris
• Flushed cheeks	• Flushed cheeks
• Heavy breathing	• Heavy breathing
• Thoughts of sex lead to a physical reaction	• Moist vagina

The Difference between Desire and Arousal

Desire or libido is the dopamine need to behave sexually in order to experience a sense of reward. It is activated by internal or external stimuli (thoughts, touch, vision, etc.), which is then adjusted by acetylcholine to create arousal: the combination of emotional attraction and cognitive attachment. Acetylcholine modifies the sexual experience so that the brain can process dopamine lust into a more human context of relationship.

acetylcholine leads to more rapid erections that occur with better blood flow.

Returning to a younger, healthier state of adequate acetylcholine levels means a moister body and a more open mind. If you have too much already, you can block it by enhancing the other brain chemicals so that you can take advantage of every sexual opportunity, instead of waiting for the perfect one.

HIGH ACETYLCHOLINE MEANS DEEP, FEELING RELATIONSHIPS

While the dopamine SexQ is all about seeking reward, acetylcholine is the key to awareness. With it, you have lots of creative ideas about keeping your sex life alive, and the ability to maintain long-lasting relationships based on fond memories. Without it, you won't be able to remember why you liked your spouse in the first place.

Most people don't have enough acetylcholine, so if you scored high on the acetylcholine part of the quiz in Chapter 3, consider yourself lucky. People with an acetylcholine SexQ are in tune with their senses. This SexQ is intuitive, which is necessary to a fulfilling sex life. You're extremely sociable, even charismatic, so people are drawn to you. When you are not in a relationship, you may find that it's very easy to find love. When you are in a relationship, you invest a great deal of energy in it. You strive to keep the romance alive.

Women with high acetylcholine SexQ know better than anyone that orgasms have more to do with the brain than the body. The feelings a woman has for her sexual partner are tied to just how good her orgasms are. A joint research project between the University of California and Geneva University studied women who were first asked to rate the ease and frequency of their orgasms compared to the quality of their relationship. These same women were given brain scans while the names of their lovers flashed before their eyes. The more "in love" the subjects judged themselves, the greater the brain activity when the name was flashed, and the higher they rated their satisfaction in their sexual relationship.

However, high acetylcholine people can constantly set themselves up for disappointment. While you understand people on a deep level, you expect others to deeply understand you. You also have perfectionist tendencies, which is where you run into trouble with your love life and your sex life, especially because life in general and your partner's specifically are rarely as perfect as you want them to be.

Lost That Lovin' Feeling?

Early symptoms of a loss of acetylcholine include memory lapses, increasing paranoia, frequent urination and bowel movements, as well as dry skin, dry vagina, low semen, and dry mouth. Before you moved rapidly from one idea to the next, one activity to another. Without acetylcholine you may find yourself obsessing on a single thought.

The goal of those with a high acetylcholine SexQ is to create balance by enhancing the other brain chemicals. More dopamine will increase your sexual desire so that you can become physical without waiting for the perfect moment. More GABA will let you relax so that you won't constantly overthink sex. And more serotonin will improve your mood so that you won't be so down on yourself when the Cinderella fantasy you were hoping for doesn't materialize.

LOW ACETYLCHOLINE MEANS GETTING BACK TO BASICS

In order to bring romance to the forefront of the sexual experience, take a step back in time and focus on foreplay. Working on your technique not only puts you back in touch with the sensual side of sex, but it is a good way to reconnect with your spouse. This means taking things a little slower and getting more creative in bed.

When men engage in foreplay, they have less anxiety about the upcoming sexual act. Foreplay helps to establish intimacy and understanding: It's essential for good, strong erections. Many men also find that prolonged foreplay enhances their orgasm, especially as they get older. Women need foreplay because it's harder for them to become aroused, and eventually orgasm, through intercourse alone.

Only you and your partner can tell when you are both truly aroused. It might take 10 minutes or it could take 2 hours. But in one 2008 study reported in the *Journal of Sexual Medicine,* thousands of Czech women of all ages reported that the average duration of foreplay was 15.4 minutes, which led to an average intercourse romp of 16.2 minutes. That's twice as long as the average American sexual encounter. If you are used to the typical American "7 minutes in heaven," think of foreplay as a brain exercise that has long-lasting effects.

Get Back to Kissing

Kissing is an essential part of foreplay. According to *Scientific American* magazine, every kiss triggers a cascade of brain signals and chemicals that "transmit tactile sensations, sexual excitement, feelings of closeness, motivation, and even euphoria."

Kisses also convey important information about the state of your relationship. Some scientists believe that kissing evolved because it so easily facilitates mate selection. That's because good kisses are addictive. Both men and women seem to enjoy even the lightest brush of the lips against any portion of their skin.

The lips themselves are among the most densely populated areas in terms of sensory neurons. When we kiss, these neurons blast messages to the brain and body, conveying both sensations and intense emotions that trigger physical reactions. Meanwhile, almost half of the cranial nerves that affect cerebral function spark, unleashing a cocktail of brain chemicals that control your levels of stress (GABA), motivation (dopamine), bonding (acetylcholine), and stimulation (serotonin).

A kiss then represents a microcosm of you and your SexQ. So if you've moved on from kissing and just get busy with the rest of sex, you and your brain are missing out.

What Else?

- **Start with a hug.** A nice, long hug (20 to 30 seconds, to be exact) has been proven to increase a woman's oxytocin level—the hormone that heightens sexual arousal.
- **Talk about what you want.** Schedule a few minutes of uninterrupted time in a relaxed setting, and sit down together to share your sexual fantasies. Let your imaginations roam free. Don't touch, just talk.
- **Take a shower together.** The sweet scents and the sexy, slippery feeling of two people in a tight, wet space have a way of moving things in the right direction.
- **Then, put your clothes back on.** Sex coach Patti Britton, PhD, says that it can be "pleasurable torture" to indulge in fully clothed foreplay, teasing and stroking your bodies through the fabric. You're building up the anticipation, so when you finally do have skin-on-skin contact, it'll be that much more explosive and exciting.
- **Or change your location.** Get out of the bedroom, pack a blanket, be discreet, and go enjoy the great outdoors!
- **Learn the art of erotic touch.** You'll need some oil and a well-heated room. Warm the oil in the palms of your hands and experiment with your partner to learn where he or she likes to be massaged.
- **Create the mood.** Aromatherapy, music, soft lighting, candles, even different textures, and revealing clothing really do alter your brain chemistry by triggering your senses. If you surround yourself with calm, with peace, for at least a portion of every day, you'll accelerate the restoration of your acetylcholine.
- **Try Allura or Zestra.** These nonprescription topical treatments are used by many women to improve sexual arousal. They can be applied to the clitoris, labia, and vaginal opening during foreplay to increase both the speed of nerve conduction and the blood flow to the genitals. It takes about 3 to 5 minutes of application and gentle massage, and its effect can last as long as 45 minutes.

Get Yourself Going

Try yoga breathing before lovemaking to increase arousal. There's no simpler way to oxygenate the blood, a process that increases sexual energy and elevates desire. Take rapid, rhythmic, and shallow breaths through the nose. Keep your mouth closed. Breathe this way for 1 to 3 minutes.

A TOY WORTH TRYING: CLITORAL PUMP

A clitoral pump is a sex toy designed for women to increase their arousal. It is often recommended by physicians for treating sexual problems connected with anorgasmia (the formal term for the inability to orgasm), because it improves blood flow to the vagina. However, this is a toy of last resort: By enhancing testosterone and oxytocin and balancing your brain chemistry, you shouldn't have to sit there and pump up your clitoris.

A clitoral pump contains a cup and a hand-squeeze bulb with a tube. The cylinder can be round or oval and is available in different sizes depending on the size of the area stimulated. It is applied to the clitoris and/or labia to create suction and may be used prior to sex or masturbation. The smaller variants are intended only for the clitoris and clitoral hood. The cylinder is placed over the clitoris, and a vacuum is created between the skin and the device by operation of the hand pump. The sucking effect makes the clitoris throb due to increased blood and skin tension. The hand pump allows complete control of the effect, and it can be stopped at any moment by releasing a valve on the tube.

IF YOU NEVER THINK ABOUT SEX, SOMETHING'S WRONG

Many of my women patients suffer from hypoactive sexual desire disorder (HSDD). This is a true medical disorder related to the loss of acetylcholine. It is defined as the persistent or recurrent absence of sexual fantasies or thoughts for and receptivity to sexual activity, which causes personal distress. When this occurs, your motivation for attempting to become sexually aroused is scarce or absent.

HSDD may occur at any time, but I find that the majority of women with this issue are between 45 and 64 years old. It may be related to menopause, but I have also found many younger women who suffer from this disorder. Some women can experience HSDD after previously experiencing an active sex life, while some women have always had low or no sexual desire.

A second type of acetylcholine disorder is classified as a sexual arousal disorder, which is limited to the physical response. Those who suffer from this have an inability to attain or maintain sufficient lubrication and vaginal swelling in response to sexual excitement.

ACETYLCHOLINE-RICH FOODS MAKE YOU FEEL SEXY

Just as you may reach for sugar and caffeine for that burst of energy to compensate for a dopamine deficiency, you might reach for rich meals, fried foods, and ice cream to self-medicate your way into thinking better and feeling sexier. An acetylcholine deficiency can make you crave foods high in fat because fat is a main source of choline, the building blocks of this brain chemical.

Eat More Vegetables for Better Sex

Antioxidants are the ultimate brain sex food because they protect the membranes of brain cells by providing building blocks for those membranes. They are common in colorful fruits and vegetables: The darker-colored choices always offer the most antioxidants. To support an acetylcholine SexQ, the best choice is asparagus, which has been shown to stop the production of acetylcholinesterase, an enzyme that destroys acetylcholine.

When you eat foods high in fat, they deliver an instant acetylcholine boost.

However, this strategy ultimately works against you. Bad fats can clog your brain and circumvent its natural mechanism for producing acetylcholine. When the brain is unable to produce acetylcholine on its own, and the fats you are feeding it aren't helping, the brain will further deplete its stores, creating an even larger deficiency.

One of the easiest ways for you to keep your acetylcholine levels balanced is by making better food choices. You'll find plenty of choline in the foods listed below. Healthy, high-choline foods also have plenty of B vitamins, which are converted through digestion to acetylcholine. Experts agree that an adequate amount of choline per day would be 425 milligrams for women and 550 milligrams for men.

Healthy Foods High in Choline

FOOD	MILLIGRAMS OF CHOLINE PER 6–8 OZ SERVING
Liver, beef	840
Liver, chicken	600
Egg (including yolk)	500
Wheat germ	300
Beef	170
Fish	160
Tofu	160
Peanuts and peanut butter	130
Almonds	100
Hazelnuts	90
Broccoli	80
Cabbage	80
Broccoli rabe	60

Foods That Arouse Your Passion

These foods have specific nutrients to boost your sex life.

Apples contain phenylethylamine (PEA), which gives you a natural feeling of well-being and excitement.

Avocado contains vitamin B$_6$, which helps to increase testosterone and potassium and regulate the thyroid gland. Both of these elements enhance libido. They also contain omega-3 fatty acids, which help the brain stay alert and focused.

Cheese contains even more PEA than chocolate does.

Chocolate contains more PEA than apples do. The darker the chocolate, the more PEA.

Nuts contain essential fatty acids that help keep the brain alert. Almonds in particular are believed to arouse passion in women. Nuts are also thought to enhance your body's own PEA, and are known to boost testosterone.

Oily fish contain omega-3 fatty acids. Found in salmon, mackerel, or trout, they make the blood less sticky, which enhances blood flow throughout the body.

You Need Lecithin for Lubrication

A second goal of an acetylcholine-balancing diet is to ensure that you have enough lecithin, a nutrient used by the body to synthesize choline. When your diet is healthy and balanced, your liver produces enough lecithin on its own. However, if your acetylcholine levels are less than ideal, you need to focus on foods that provide this vital nutrient.

Only a limited number of foods contain sufficient amounts of lecithin, so if you are acetylcholine deficient, you'll need to work these into your diet.

- Cauliflower
- Egg yolks
- Liver
- Milk
- Peanuts
- Soybeans
- Wheat germ

Spices Arouse More Than Your Taste Buds

Turmeric is literally the spice of life, because it stimulates the production of acetylcholine, and it has been proved to help unclog amyloid, the garbage that mucks up the pathways of the brain. Without amyloid, your thinking is much clearer. These other spices are all known to improve your sex life, and your acetylcholine levels.

- Allspice
- Basil
- Cumin
- Peppermint
- Sage
- Thyme
- Turmeric

NUTRIENTS THAT ENCOURAGE AROUSAL

Acetylcholine supplements are brain-speed boosting; they are best taken a half hour before eating, in the early morning through the afternoon, to keep you sharp during the day. Acetylcholine may be an important brain chemical in the regulation of penile erections, so anything that increases acetylcholine may improve erections. Many of these nutrients are precursors to acetylcholine, so they should essentially lead to the same thing—improved erections.

While you don't need a doctor's prescription to buy these, you do need to know how they will affect your health, especially if you have already been diagnosed with chronic illness or disease. Discuss all of these options with your doctor, and choose together which ones may be best for you. Most will also improve your memory as well as your current health status and your sexual function.

NATURAL TREATMENTS	SUGGESTED DAILY DOSAGE	HOW IT AFFECTS SEX
Acetyl-L-Carnitine	500–5,000 mg	This nutrient and its relative propionyl-L-carnitine may be more effective than testosterone for improving erections. Also is thought to improve memory, heart disease, and liver cleansing.
Choline	200–3,000 mg	Precursor to acetylcholine. May increase sexual desire in people over 40 years old. May improve erections, as well as memory, concentration, attention.
Dimethylaminoethanol (DMAE)	100–3,000 mg	May increase sexual desire, allow for better erections, and improve memory.
Fish Oil (omega-3)	500–3,000 mg	Improves circulation, which helps with erections. Is also used to treat arthritis, heart disease, blood pressure, and inflammatory issues.
GPC (Glycerophosphoryl-choline)	200–1,000 mg	May improve mood by increasing dopamine levels, and improve erections by increasing acetylcholine levels. A good choice if choline doesn't work for you.
Phosphatidyl Serine	100–300 mg	May improve mood by increasing dopamine levels, and improve erections by increasing acetylcholine levels. Also thought to improve memory and attention.
Piracetam (derivative of GABA)	2,000–5,000 mg	Works well with choline, which may lead to better erections and reverse memory loss.

ESTROGEN REVERSES EVERYTHING, INCLUDING YOUR SexQ

Estrogen is produced primarily in the ovaries, but it is also produced in both men and women in the skin, brain, bone, vascular system, and breast tissue.

Estrogen keeps the brain young by stimulating acetylcholine production. However, as we age and lose acetylcholine, we also lose the ability to create estrogen. In women, menopause occurs as a result of this significant change in hormone levels. This can affect cognitive function (brain speed) as well as sexual arousal (internal lubrication), which is why vaginal dryness and pain during intercourse are associated not only with declining acetylcholine but with a lowering of estrogen. By the age of 30, most women are entering perimenopause, the earliest stages of estrogen decline, and need some additional natural estrogen to increase lubrication so that they can become aroused.

Bioidentical Estrogen Options

- **Bi-est:** oral capsules and topical gels
- **Estradiol:** sublingual, percutaneous, or transdermal "Vivelle Dot" patch
- **Tri-est:** oral capsules and topical gels
- **Vagifem:** inserted into the vagina to help with lubrication and strengthen vaginal area
- **Viafem:** a great supplement, not a prescription; it's so effective that I call it "scream cream"

Women who continue to enjoy sex as they age typically have more estrogen and subsequently feel "younger." Estrogen helps maintain the condition of the vaginal lining and its elasticity, and it produces vaginal lubrication. I have found that bioidentical estrogen replacement may be helpful in treating vaginal atrophy, decreasing pain during intercourse, and improving clitoral sensitivity. In men, estrogen levels decrease slowly. Supplementing lost estrogen is thought to work in conjunction with testosterone to increase lustful desire.

The quiz in Chapter 3 can help alert you to the earliest possible losses of estrogen. When this happens, we need to build estrogen levels back through natural sex-hormone-replacement therapies, diet, and nutrient supplementation. You'll learn more about menopause and estrogen replacement therapies in Chapter 8.

Case Study: Janine's Lack of Arousal Was the Result of an Underlying Condition

Janine came to see me because all of a sudden, she couldn't concentrate. After a brain checkup, I realized that she had developed adult attention deficit disorder at 40 years old. I prescribed Adderall and acetylcholine-boosting supplements, and when she came back a month later, her whole demeanor had changed. Not only had her ability to

Dead Nipple Syndrome

I recently treated a woman who uses her nipples as her sexual barometer: When her nipples are erect, she is ready for sex. But all of a sudden, they weren't "working," and neither was her sex life. I told her that she had dead nipple syndrome. But once she started on the Braverman Protocol, she was able to increase her arousal by raising her GABA, serotonin, and acetylcholine levels with natural estrogen cream that she put right on her nipples. Within a few weeks, her nipples turned on again and so did she.

focus improved, so had her sex life. The Adderall increased her desire, and the supplements increased her arousal. She told me that this was the best side effect from medications that she ever had.

Whenever you have to use medicine, you can enhance its effect when you supplement it with nutrients that correspond to the medication's brain chemical augmentation. In this way you'll be getting the proverbial "biggest bang for the buck," because you will be increasing all aspects of a heightened brain chemistry. In this case, Janine increased her arousal when her acetylcholine was amplified, even though she was treating her ADD. Now that's the kind of side effect everyone can enjoy.

ACETYLCHOLINE MEDICATIONS

The following medications are currently prescribed to work with acetylcholine to increase erection ability and sex drive. Discuss them with your doctor to determine if they are necessary, and if they will affect other health issues you may be experiencing.

- Viagra, Levitra, Cialis: increase vascular blood flow (see Chapter 10)
- Dementia medications such as Aricept, Namenda, Exelon, Prostigmin, Tacrine, and Reminyl: increase sex drive

WHEN YOU'RE THINKING, YOU CAN THINK ABOUT SEX

Keeping your brain constantly engaged is one of the keys to staying younger and sexier. By keeping up with the world around you, as well as your personal life, you are stimulating acetylcholine production as you increase your intellect. And as you exercise your brain, you are increasing its ability for attention and retention, therefore creating more "brain memory." So continue reading books, magazines, or the newspaper, completing word or number puzzles, engaging in intellectual conversation, or even creating artwork. Not only will you be more fun at cocktail parties, you'll be more fun in bed. That's because a quick-thinking, high acetylcholine brain is worth 15 more years of great sex.

Lastly, start thinking about yourself in a more positive light. Compared with the entire world's population, there are very few supermodels or professional athletes walking around. Don't create an expectation where those exceptional people determine how you should look or feel about yourself. For most of us, those are not achievable goals and shouldn't become another reason for not having sex. Sadly, a 2005 study reported at the International Society for the Study of Women's Sexual Health showed that 94 percent of women and 63 percent of men agreed with the statement, "If I am feeling unattractive, it is harder for me to get sexually aroused." So do yourself and your spouse a favor: If they tell you that they love you just the way you are, believe them and show them that you love them for feeling that way.

CHAPTER 6

GABA Makes Sex Your Ally

HALF OF THE world's population is GABA dominant. While that means it's easy to find a partner that is "just like you," this SexQ is responsible for creating and upholding many negative sexual stereotypes. GABA men may think that married women are done with sex, and they might be right. GABA women find that men just need sex more than women, and there is some truth to that statement as well. But as you are learning, your life doesn't have to be defined by these statements. You can create a better, more active sex life for you and your spouse, one that brings you closer together emotionally as well as physically. When you learn to make sex your ally, you'll find that it helps you reexamine every aspect of your life. And you can accomplish this just by enhancing your brain chemistry.

The chemical family that controls the brain's and the body's pace is known as GABA, which stands for gamma-amino butyric acid. GABA is produced in the temporal lobes and is delivered as calming, rhythmic waves. GABA controls the brain's pace and the communication between the brain and the body: It keeps all the other electrical sparks and brain chemicals in check. By monitoring your internal rhythm, GABA has a calming, stabilizing effect over the brain and the body. Unlike dopamine and acetylcholine, GABA and serotonin are the electrical "off" switches: They inhibit communication in the brain, which helps you slow down, regroup, relax, and sleep. GABA prevents us from overreacting, or getting "too juiced." While that's helpful in the boardroom, it's not the best in the bedroom.

There's nothing wrong with a GABA SexQ, but it is perhaps the most stuck in its ways. That's because a GABA brain is an organized brain. In your home, it's quite likely that everything has its place, and the same holds true for the roles you play in your marriage or relationship. You love schedules because they eliminate the worry about uncertainty. Sex for you may be Wednesday nights after the kids go to sleep or Saturday nights after your big "date night." You may enjoy sex and you may not. You may orgasm, but it's likely that you don't, and don't really care. You derive your pleasure from the fulfillment of obligation and taking care of those you love.

This is not the way healthy, younger, loving sex is supposed to be. GABA has been your bonding ally, but it's time to shake things up. High GABA people become too connected to commitment, and for many, when commitment goes up, sexuality goes down, and they have to get out of that rut. Otherwise, they're so committed to each other that they become sexually paralyzed by duty, and they can't have any fun. So if your sex life is so predictable—10:05 p.m. in a missionary position—you must learn a wider variety of sexual responses so that your brain also has increased creativity. Most relationships won't be able to sustain unspoken sexual boredom or tension.

Younger sex is less organized sex. It's not about your obligation to your spouse; it's more about creating intimacy. Your life doesn't have to be defined by what you are doing for someone else. You are not doing anyone a "favor" by engaging in compulsory, lifeless sex. In fact, you'll be much better at taking care of others once you learn how to be more sexually engaged. And that means truly letting go in every aspect of your life.

I promise that if you can balance your GABA and boost your other brain chemi-cals, you'll become a little more "turned on" and a lot less "turned off." You will feel more intuitive and have a lot more desire. Better still, you'll find that you are less codependent, less addicted to overnurturing because you've gained in bed. You'll be better at every aspect of your life, and you will feel younger and sexier, which is the ultimate commitment that you can make to yourself and your spouse.

THE GABA PARADOX

When GABA is unbalanced, you become unbalanced. You can feel overly emotional and mentally or physically rocky; you might be nervous, tense, or irritable, even hungry. It becomes difficult to relax and let go during sex. Anxiety kills sex: You will not be able to have an orgasm if you are tense. You can also develop a complete indifference to sex. High GABA people report that they are sick of sex: They are bored of it, think "it's dumb," and they remove themselves from the physical act entirely. They feel trapped by commitment, but don't know what to do about it. High GABA women, in particular, can't let go of their spouse or partner. Lowering GABA allows women who consider sexual fantasies taboo to explore their sexual desires.

GABA levels need to be just right in order to create perfect marital bonding and achieve orgasm. In fact, too much human bonding and commitment inter-feres with creative sexuality. It's the human paradox. In order to have a more balanced SexQ, you might need to let go of some of your protective commitment and have some fun.

Fetishes, Tourette's Syndrome, and Obsessive-Compulsive Behaviors

Figuring out what turns you on is the first half of what great sex is all about. And if you recognize that you need a little help in order to orgasm, whether from sex toys or special requests, then more power to you. I'm hoping that when you balance your brain, your reliance on these will diminish.

The term *fetish* refers to a sexual attraction to something that is not traditionally considered sexually arousing. It can be anything from objects, materials, or body parts that simply aren't deemed sexual by the rest of society. For some people, sexual arousal is impossible without the fetish object.

A fetish is generally considered a problem only when it interferes with normal functioning outside the sexual arena, such as exposing genitals to strangers, rubbing against strangers, and child obsessions. Milder fetishes include an attachment to certain fabrics or types of clothing, lying, giving or receiving pain, urination, erotic talk, body piercing, voyeurism, cross-dressing, suffocating, filth obsessions, and using animals. All are signals that you are stuck on one thought: a true GABA imbalance.

Obsessive-compulsive disorders and Tourette's syndrome are also signs of an anxious GABA brain. People with obsessive-compulsive disorder often overlap with those who suffer from Tourette's syndrome: Both display uncontrollable urges and unusual sexual behaviors. I have written several papers with David Comings, MD, a specialist in this field, who notes that families plagued by Tourette's syndrome often suffer from other unusual behavior, including violence and abuse. However, with proper medications that rebalance GABA, as well as antidepressants like Zoloft, Prozac, Effexor, Celexa, and Lexapro, these sexual and otherwise bizarre symptoms can and will diminish.

GABA Balances a High Dopamine SexQ

A person with a high dopamine and high acetylcholine SexQ lusts for a combination of conquest and romance but is able to suppress feelings of intimacy—a deadly combination in the dating world. This histrionic, attention-seeking drama-queen/drama-prince lifestyle so many politicians display is nothing more than brain chemistry excess: They are craving and addicted to variety in their relationships. They never stop to think how this addictive behavior is an irrational risk that will ultimately damage their children, their families, and their lives.

The good news is that you now have the tools to create better awareness. And with these you can learn to harness the one brain chemical that can offset boundary issues to rebalance your SexQ: GABA saves men and women from sexual scandal.

Too Much GABA Leaves Little Room for You

A brain that produces too much GABA has ratcheted up nurturing tendencies. These people spend their entire lives looking for love and opportunities to give care at the suffocating expense of being hurt because their needs are never met. They rely heavily on their mates and authority figures for advice. Cult leaders prey on these types of people because they just do what they're told.

With too much GABA, you've given in, and you've given up. Sex has become a pain: It's either too messy or truly physically painful. *Dyspareunia* is the medical term for painful or uncomfortable intercourse, for both men and women. High GABA women may also experience pain in their breasts and pain to the touch of their skin.

Ironically, high GABA women are often attracted to high dopamine men. On one hand, they like to be told what to do. On the other, they become turned off by the constant requests for sex. You can dial down your GABA by dialing up your sex life to meet the needs of your spouse, if you want to.

More dopamine will increase your sex drive, making you and your partner a better sexual match. More acetylcholine will put you back in touch with—or creates from scratch—your romantic side, which will put you in the mood. More serotonin will make sex fun, so you'll look forward to having some.

When You're Tense, You Lose Your Intensity

A balanced brain creates and receives electricity in a smooth, even flow. When your brain is not producing enough GABA, your brain's electricity is generated in bursts. This is called a brain arrhythmia,

Your Sex Life Suffers When You're Married to Your Job

GABA people are the most dependable. You can be counted on to show up every day to do your job and to be there when others need you. But if you are giving, giving, giving all day long, you're exhausted at night, and you simply don't have the energy for sex. The key to a better brain, and a better sex life, is balance. Pace yourself during the day; don't be the one who always "gives at the office" so that you can give more to your spouse in the bedroom.

or dysrhythmia, and it can upset your physical and emotional life in a variety of ways. When your rhythm is affected by a GABA deficiency, you may begin to feel anxious, nervous, or irritable because the communication in your brain is like constant chatter. You're stressed about the big things in life, but you can't let go of the details, either. You may complain more regularly that you don't feel well, or you may develop a chronic pain that never goes away. You're uncomfortable in your own skin.

There is no way that you can relax when it comes to sex, and orgasm is nearly impossible or not as intense as it used to be (the medical term *anorgasmia* refers to regular difficulty reaching orgasm after ample sexual stimulation). You may not want to have sex at all because the prospect of sex produces fear or anxiety (sexual aversion disorder). You may experience either increased or decreased sensitivity in your genitals upon physical stimulation. At the same time, you are hypersexual, sexually frustrated with your intense desire for sex without the ability to perform. Women can experience involuntary vaginal contractions that prevent vaginal penetration (the medical term is *vaginismus,* but I call this a vagina panic attack). Men can experience weaker erections, decreased strength, decreased endurance, performance anxiety, or require more stimuli than before to achieve an erection,

> ## GABA Sexual Archetypes
>
> The list of high GABA archetypes is endless and includes anyone who's been left in the dust by a famous spouse. The media makes a big deal out of their dalliances, but the writing was always on the wall.
>
> **Too much:** Catherine of Aragon—Henry XIII's first wife, who refused to divorce her husband
>
> **Too little:** Michael Jackson—the ultimate wunderkind who could never come to terms with adult relationships, sexual or otherwise

or what I call numb penis syndrome. This results in painful orgasm/ejaculation or erectile constipation because the sufferer is not relaxed enough to let go. All of these conditions can be primary ("I've never been able to") or secondary ("I used to be able to but can't anymore") as well as situational ("I can achieve orgasm when I masturbate but not with partners," for example).

So you put sex off for another night, hoping your spouse won't notice. But they do, and they're not happy about it.

SIGNS OF A LOW GABA SexQ:

- Some part of my body always hurts when I have sex.
- I'm too embarrassed to enjoy sex.
- I'd rather eat than have sex.
- I share too much personal information about my life with others.
- I'm nervous and jumpy.
- My thoughts get too confused.

IS ANXIETY AFFECTING YOUR SEX LIFE?

Stress can get the better of all of us, but when you have a GABA SexQ, you suffer the most. That's because the brain can create a vicious stress loop that's hard to break. In a 2009 article appearing in the journal *Science,* researchers at the Life and Health Sciences Research Institute at the University of Minho, in Portugal, found that the sensation of being highly stressed can rewire the brain to promote its persistence. Their experiments with laboratory rats revealed that chronically stressed rats lost their cunning and instead resorted to familiar routines and rote responses, like compulsively pressing a bar for food pellets even though they weren't hungry. When their brains were more closely observed, it was found that the dopamine regions associated with executive decision making and goal-directed behaviors had shriveled, while the GABA sectors linked to habit formation had bloomed. The stressed rats were now cognitively conditioned to keep doing the same things over and over instead of trying something new. They couldn't break their own vicious cycle.

This may show one of the reasons why when you get stressed, you follow the same loop. Either you eat way too much or simply complain incessantly. Or you find yourself in the "no sex" rut, the "no intimacy" rut, or the "no orgasm" rut. Wherever you end up, I guarantee it isn't sexy.

Sexual stress, or performance anxiety, increases cortisol levels, which decreases GABA. This means that you can't calm down, no matter how hard you try. The key is to boost your GABA before engaging in sexual relations, so that you'll be calm from the beginning.

Luckily, an overstressed brain, just like any other physical or mental condition, is reversible. We can learn better ways to handle stress. For one, great, orgasmic sex can help us release some of the stress of the day and break the stress cycle, which is why you need to make sex your ally. Best of all, a life without anxiety is worth 10 more years of great sex.

First, figure out what you are stressed about. Then determine how to incorporate more, better sex into your life so that you can relax and step off the hamster wheel of stress.

The Whole Body Suffers from Stress

- Blood pressure increases
- Arteries stiffen
- Immune system shuts down
- Risk of diabetes increases
- Risk of depression increases
- Risk of Alzheimer's disease increases
- Risk of heart disease increases
- Risk of obesity increases
- Sleeplessness increases

THE TOO-STRESSED-FOR-SEX TEST

Sometimes you know what's on your mind, and other times you are too far into the rut to recognize the initial problem. Take a quick look over your average day and see what's stressing you out.

IS IT THE JOB?

- Do you have problems with your commute time or related issues?
- Is your job satisfying?
- Are you currently working on a difficult project or deadline?
- Are the people in your office difficult to deal with?

IS IT THE FAMILY?

- Are you spending enough (or too much) time with your children?
- If your family life satisfying?
- Has there been a recent family event/illness/divorce/move that you are dealing with?
- Is money (too much or lack of) creating problems within your family?

IS IT YOUR RELATIONSHIPS?

- Are you spending enough (or too much) time with your spouse/partner?
- Are you spending enough (or too much) time within a social network?
- Are you happy with your friends and community?
- Has there been a recent event/illness/divorce/move within your community that involves you directly or tangentially?

ARE YOU HAPPY WITH YOURSELF?

- Are you making time for exercise?
- Are you making time for fun/recreation?
- Are you engaged in spiritual activities or community?
- Are you engaged in frequent, loving sex?

Where Did the Love Go?

In most marriages, the honeymoon period doesn't last, and once-hot-and-sweaty sex "matures" into something deeper, more meaningful. Or the relationship just disappears. The question is why? Does sex become boring, or does something happen to the brain and the body that makes us less excited by those we love?

Stressed about Sex

If sex is the thing that's stressing you out, talk about it with your partner. Remember, there are no rules. You shouldn't be ashamed of the number of sexual partners you've had (great or small), your range of desire, or your lack or wealth of sexual knowledge. As long as what you want to do in bed is safe and consensual, don't create anxiety around it.

It turns out to be a little of both. Studies have shown many different causes for the lost sexual spark of marriage, including the addition of children into the family, changes in daily living, and a changing perspective or worldview. And that's not even considering an aging brain or aging body.

Younger sex is hot, sweaty, frequent, and deeply committed. That's what I want for you. There's no reason that you have to act "mature" in the bedroom, when what your brain really needs is a little bit of wildness in order to reset for faster thinking, healthier living, and better loving.

Case Study: Paula Reversed 17 Years Without Sex

Doctors used to think that the inability to achieve orgasm by intercourse alone was such a sufficiently common problem that it was not regarded as a dysfunction. Luckily, we now know better. You can—and should—achieve orgasms, regardless of your age. In fact, you are entitled to younger, more frequent sex whether you are 27 or 77. If you are not enjoying sex, something is wrong with your brain chemistry, and you might have to try something new.

Paula was 63 years old when she became my patient and confided that she was only having sex four times a year. In 1986 her husband had started taking high blood pressure medication, which slowly caused erectile dysfunction, and therefore eliminated his sex drive and her sex life. For the next

17 years their marriage continued with only the most infrequent sexual activity, until the couple came to see me.

"I first came to see Dr. Braverman when I was 63, and the sex issue was discussed in our very first visit. He told us that a healthy sex life should include some sexual activity at least three times a week. At that time Viagra had just come out in the marketplace, and he prescribed it for my husband, along with testosterone supplementation. When we did my physical, we discovered that I had no estrogen or testosterone in my body; I had already gone through menopause 13 years prior. Dr. Braverman put me on bioidentical estrogens, testosterone, and progesterone. Then we had a frank talk about our sex life. He made a few suggestions and told us to come back in a month to see how we responded to his protocol."

The next time the couple came into my office, Paula was obviously pleased. She told me almost immediately that while she was comfortable having her husband take Viagra once a week, she was still afraid that too much sex would kill him. Best of all, she had taken my advice to heart: They were trying something new. Once a week they would have sex, and on other days her husband would perform oral sex on her. Now she is having four orgasms a week—what she considers to be the best sex of her life!

"We both responded quickly to his therapies. I am now 69 years old, and the sex is still the best ever. I put the testosterone cream on my clitoris every night before bed. Oral sex is out of this world, and the endorphins that are created in the brain keep me happy the entire next day. No woman has lived a full life if she has not felt this kind of pleasure."

Paula and I agree that each of us only has one life to enjoy here on earth. So I was more than pleased to hear that she feels the best she ever has. She is the happiest she has ever been and would love time to stop right now so that she can continue to feel this way forever.

THE BIOLOGY OF ORGASM

Scientists are still researching whether orgasm is the consequence of biological mechanics or if it is primarily a brain phenomenon. We know they are intimately connected, because the brain has been imaged during orgasm using functional MRIs (fMRI), PET scans, and BEAM technology. These images clearly show that your brain's health is at the core of your sexual health.

Orgasm is a multisensory experience that involves the entire person—mind and body. Studies have shown that those who have suffered from stroke or brain trauma have decreased ability for sexual activity, while those who have experienced spinal cord injuries can continue to have pleasurable sexual responses in different parts of the body. What's more, the latest brain research shows that sexual functioning, including desire, motivation, anxiety, orgasm, ejaculation, and pleasure, is jointly determined by the genitals as well as the brain's peripheral and central neural pathways. The mind

component includes not only the emotional attachment that occurs during sex, but the sexual component as well. Physically, sensory fields in the genitals and skin are directly connected to nerves and react upon stimulation. This means that sensations in the genitals are governed by your head. If you think that you can get away with bad brain chemistry and still have great orgasms, forget it.

A woman's orgasm is usually achieved from continuous stimulation of any of the following: the clitoris, vagina, cervix, breasts, or nipples. Every woman is different, and each will respond to touch differently. But whatever works causes the brain to release oxytocin from the pituitary gland into the bloodstream at four times more than normal levels. Muscle contractions then begin at the pelvic floor, the uterus, and the vagina. At the same time, the labia and clitoris become engorged with blood. Blood pressure and heart rate double their resting levels. There is also a noticeable reduction in the response to pain, although sensitivity to touch increases. In the brain, areas that control thoughts and emotions are shut down temporarily; this may correspond to a release of tension and inhibition.

For men, arousal activates the parasympathetic or involuntary nerves that extend from the pelvic region of the spinal cord and end in an area of the penis called the corpora cavernosum. The penis tissue becomes filled with blood to produce an erection. The nerves are stimulated by the release of oxytocin-filled neurons that originated in the brain. The nerves then release nitric oxide and acetylcholine, as well as other chemicals and hormones, which relax the involuntary muscles of the penis and allow for increased blood flow. The brain's center of vigilance shuts down. Ejaculation follows, with the rhythmical expulsion of semen. At this point, blood is no longer flowing toward the penis tissue. This is called detumescence.

Both men and women describe orgasm with similar language. It is identified as a feeling of tension building and then a release that is both pleasurable and exciting. The orgasm is both the highest point of tension and the release almost at the same time.

Orgasms Are the Intention of Intercourse

If you are waiting for sex to be "over with," you're never going to have an orgasm. You may need to slow things down and hold back on penetration in order to build up intimacy, establishing more of an acetylcholine SexQ. The following exercises are meant to slow down lovemaking so that you can focus on your partner physically and emotionally. Just as the foreplay exercises in Chapter 5 let you reacquaint yourself with your lover, these exercises are meant to create an open dialogue where you can discuss what turns you on and off. This can include various sexual positions as well as personality issues, or even positive or negative aspects of your day. When you

work on rekindling the love in your relationship—the art of daily living as well as your compatible worldview—then you'll really feel the love in bed.

The first set of exercises that I prescribe doesn't focus on orgasm at all. Instead, the intention is to re-create the loving aspects of your relationship without the pressure of climax. The first exercise is called karezza, which is similar to another sexual exercise known as coitus reservatus (but not coitus interruptus, which is the withdrawal method of birth control). Both of these techniques involve sexual intercourse in which the man does not attempt to ejaculate within his partner, but instead remains at the plateau phase of intercourse for as long as possible, avoiding the orgasm and seminal emission. The technique is meant to prolong sexual pleasure for both the man and the woman. The goal is to separate orgasm from ejaculation for men, and orgasm from climax for women, and being able to identify and experience one without the other.

Karezza is a form of extended physical and emotional foreplay, an arousing and effective method to intensify the desire of sexual pleasure within the context of long-term relationships. One of the prerequisites of karezza is to have less sex, not more, and to build up levels of communication between the couple over the weeks it takes the body to fully recover from each orgasm. When you do have sex, I suggest that you try to make love slowly and gently, to relax rather than suppress orgasm, and to be mindful of each partner's state of arousal and attentive to your own breathing.

Coitus reservatus is a technique that can be practiced more frequently. During this exercise, women enjoy a prolonged orgasm while the man demonstrates complete self-control. This exercise is particularly useful when the woman is the one with the sexual difficulty.

Another technique of orgasm control is known as peaking, which is defined as a sexual act where an active partner (or giver) takes control over a passive partner's (or receiver's) orgasm. The giver sexually stimulates the receiver, gradually bringing them up to a point very high in the plateau phase where an orgasm is actually building, and will then reduce the level of stimulation just below that needed to trigger the orgasm. By carefully varying the intensity of stimulation, the receiver is held in a highly aroused state. Repetition of this process can create an overwhelming urge to orgasm. Both partners can trade roles. The partner with the sexual difficulty can be either the giver or the receiver. Sometimes, fully understanding another person's orgasm will help unleash your own.

A TOY WORTH TRYING: VIBRATOR

Vibrators are small electric appliances that are often recommended by doctors and sex therapists for people who have difficulty reaching orgasm by other means. Couples also use them as an enhancement to the pleasure of one or both partners. Some vibrators are marketed as "body massagers." Some run on batteries while others have a power cord that plugs into a wall socket.

Orgasms can occur outside of genital stimulation. For example, many people have orgasms in their sleep or by stimulating nongenital parts of the body with the use of a vibrator. That's why it is a misconception that vibrators are only for women. While it's true that vibrators can help women achieve orgasm, they can also provide great stimulation on the head, shaft, and base of the penis, as well as the testicles. Some men use a vibrator to massage the area underneath the scrotum. Vibrators can help some men who can't maintain a full erection to have an orgasm.

There is a wide range of styles, sizes, and particular features among vibrators. Some even play music! Whatever you choose to try is your personal preference. Don't let your partner, or even a friend, make you feel bad about exploring this option for orgasm.

The Skills of a Great Lover

A great lover is a patient lover. On average it takes women almost 20 minutes to achieve an orgasm, while a man can climax in just 6. So if you're a woman in a rush, you'll lose the race to good sex every time.

Once time is on your side, let's look at the way you've been having sex lately. For instance, the most traditional position, the missionary, is the least likely bodily alignment to bring a woman to climax. But if your GABA SexQ allows no room for change, then there is a subtle adjustment you can make that can increase your chances of having an orgasm. It's called the coital alignment technique, or CAT.

While you are lying on your back, have your partner move his entire body up about 2 inches. Your partner's pubic bone will rest on top of yours so that the base of his penis presses on your clitoris. This position provides continuous stimulation of your clitoris during intercourse, increasing your chances of having an orgasm.

The GABA SexQ likes sex the same way, every time. I recommend switching things up as much as possible to see what really turns you and your partner on. Over the course of a relationship, you will probably have sex thousands of times: What do you think is sexy about doing it the same way every single time? Consult the Kama Sutra or any popular magazine to learn dozens of sexual positions. At least three of them should be right for you.

Learning to Love Touch

When you have a balanced brain and can learn to let go of some GABA control, you'll find that you will enjoy being touched. Lots of people enjoy nonaggressive touching or caressing of their hair, ears, eyelids, nose, neck, upper back, lower back, breast, chest, belly, genitals, butt, thighs, legs, and feet. Others can be trained to enjoy touch. Touch is critical to resetting your GABA SexQ and developing good GABA skills. Not only do you have to learn to be able to be touched by others, but you have to be able to touch every part of your own body.

The Fabled G-Spot Is Easy to Find

The G-spot was named in 1981 for gynecologist Ernst Grafenberg, who first described the erogenous zone in 1950. Men and women have been looking for it ever since. You can find yours, or your partner's, on the front wall of the vagina, usually about a third of the way up from the vaginal opening. This area is surrounded by erectile tissues and made up of a cluster of glands surrounding the urethra, called Skene's glands. During stimulation, the urethra will enlarge and the G-spot can be easily located. Continued touch will likely produce orgasm. Sometimes, orgasm will occur along with female ejaculate, a fluid chemically similar to semen. Many women mistake this sudden wetness for urinary incontinence. Women should also know that this experience is not uncommon. In one study printed in the *Journal of Sex Research,* 40 percent of the women in the study reported experiencing female ejaculation.

The G-spot can be stimulated by the penis or with your partner's finger (when you're facing each other) by making a beckoning "come here" motion inside the vagina. Other people find that vibrators are more effective. You'll know when you have hit the spot, because you will feel a strong urge to urinate, but don't stop.

If, despite your best attempts, you are unable to achieve a G-spot orgasm, don't despair: It may be due to anatomy rather than lack of effort. Some women have little

Sex Begets Better Sex

Women don't have to have a high dopamine SexQ or a high acetylcholine SexQ in order to have good sex. Sometimes, good sex will come regardless, as long as it's consensual.

This means that you don't have to wait for the moment to be right or put off sex if you don't feel like it. It just might happen that once you've been asked and become engaged, you're able to relax and enjoy the moment. This is the real GABA lesson.

to no prostatic tissue in the vagina, which means that there is nothing to stimulate. It is estimated that about 15 percent of women are affected in this way, but you won't know if you are one of them unless you try.

GET MORE GABA FOODS FOR BETTER ORGASMS

Anxiety and frigidity can be solved by balancing GABA. The easiest and most natural way for you to keep your GABA balanced is with the foods you eat. The goal of a GABA diet is to ensure that the body has enough raw materials—in this case complex carbohydrates—for creating a steady supply of glutamine, the amino acid that is the precursor to GABA. This allows the body's natural processes to function and keeps your mood stable.

Inositol and B Vitamins Let You Relax

Inositol is a vitamin in the B-complex family that is also related to GABA. Foods

Foods High in Glutamine and Inositol

FOOD	MILLIGRAMS PER 6–8 OZ SERVING
Brown rice	940
Whole grains	860
Potatoes	830
Halibut	790
Broccoli	740
Spinach	680
Beef liver and other organ meats	650
Tree nuts	540
Rice bran	370
Lentils	280
Banana	220
Citrus fruits	210

Foods for Thought

Figs contain magnesium, which is a great agent for soothing nerves and augmenting GABA. Cherries contain anthocyanins which can help lower inflammation, making you more comfortable and in a better mood for sex.

that feature inositol can help you feel calm and relaxed by activating GABA. The more GABA-producing and GABA-enhancing foods you eat, the more GABA you will be able to create. The Bs—bananas, broccoli, and brown rice—are all packed with inositol.

A Spicy Meal Calms the Brain

Generous use of these spices can provide relief when you are stressed and can alleviate complaints that lead you to avoid having sex. For instance, rosemary can ward off headaches because it helps keep blood vessels dilated (also good for sex). Sage can help lessen menopausal night sweats, helping you to relax.

- Caraway
- Cardamom
- Cilantro
- Cinnamon
- Cloves
- Coriander
- Lemongrass
- Oregano
- Paprika
- Poppy seeds
- Rosemary
- Sage

Wine Makes You Feel Younger and Sexier

Most everyone's vision of a romantic evening involves a bottle of wine. But why wine more than any other alcoholic beverage? Alcohol in general increases GABA levels, which makes you feel more relaxed. But wine—and especially red wine—has the added benefit of being a great source of the antioxidant resveratrol, which helps open the arteries by enhancing the body's ability to produce nitric oxide. This chemical forces the blood vessels to expand, which allows more blood to travel to the genitals, increasing arousal. Red wine also contains aromatase inhibitors, which allow testosterone to convert safely to estrogen, ramping up any libido.

Make sure you stop at one or two glasses—too much alcohol makes for a restless night. A man won't be able to maintain an erection, and a woman could go right to sleep. Alcohol suppresses deep sleep, causing sleep fragmentation and contributing to sleep apnea. Alcohol also depresses testosterone levels, which means you're less likely to be in the right mood later in the evening.

Recreational Drugs Are Always a Bad Idea

Marijuana, like alcohol, helps people relax enough to reach orgasm. The drug known as Ecstasy increases sociability and generates positive feelings toward sex. Amyl nitrite, or "poppers," when taken at the moment of orgasm, is thought to increase its intensity. Amphetamines and cocaine can increase sexual stamina. Yet in the long run, all of these party drugs do more harm than good, damaging your brain and requiring escalating and more frequent dosages.

There's no point in creating an unnecessary addiction, especially to something that is hazardous to your health. That's why the GABA-enhancing techniques covered in this chapter are so important: You can use proven therapies to become more present in your sexuality, and find greater intimacy without the negative side effects of illegal drugs or alcohol.

Case Study: Susan and Freddie Were Way Too GABA

Susan and Freddie were high school sweethearts who had been married for 20 years when they came to see me. Unfortunately, their sex life was still connected to their party lifestyle. The only times they were able to have satisfying sex were when they were both completely drunk. While this worked for them, the calories were adding up: Both were on the border of obesity, and Susan had just received a "pre-diabetes" warning from her doctor. She was resigned to reducing the sugar in her diet, but she wasn't willing to let go of the wine—and the last vestiges of their youthful sex life.

I was able to show this couple other solutions to their sexual problems. First, they had to recognize that their SexQ wasn't healthy. Then, I put them on the modified amino acid taurine to cut their alcohol craving. I also prescribed a mild testosterone cream they could both use—at different dosages—to give their sex drive a jump start. It took them a while to give up the alcohol completely, but they were able to let it go once they realized it was no longer an essential part of their sex life.

VITAMINS AND SUPPLEMENTS THAT KEEP YOU CONNECTED

Vitamins and supplements are an excellent way to ensure a steady supply of GABA nutrients. Taken in the late afternoon or early evening, they will help you relax and unwind. While these nutrients won't improve your ability to orgasm, they will relax the brain so that you feel less anxious and more confident, which is integral to better sex.

While you don't need a doctor's prescription to buy these, you do need to know how they will affect your health, especially if you have already been diagnosed with chronic illness or disease. Discuss all of

NATURAL TREATMENTS	SUGGESTED DAILY DOSAGE	HOW IT AFFECTS SEX
GABA	500–3,000 mg	Controls anxiety
Inositol	500–10,000 mg	Produces a calming and relaxing effect
Magnesium	300–1,000 mg	May help with premature ejaculation. Also used to reverse heart disease and constipation.
Melatonin	0.5–5 mg	May help with impotence, improve sexual performance, and help with sleep.
Taurine	500–10,000 mg	Increases GABA levels in the brain. Used to treat high blood pressure, gall bladder conditions, and alcoholism.
Theanine	100–500 mg	Increases GABA levels in the brain. Reduces mental and physical stress and may produce feelings of relaxation. Used to treat anxiety and high blood pressure.
Valerian root	200–400 mg	Inhibits the breakdown of GABA. Used to treat sleep disorders and anxiety attacks.
Vitamin B_6	10–100 mg	May improve sexual performance, as well as enhance serenity and relaxation after sex. Is used to treat depression and inadequate dream recall.

these options with your doctor, and choose together which ones may be best for you. Read carefully to see if they will improve your current health status as well as your ability to relax and let go.

Teas Calm an Anxious Brain

Research has shown that L-theanine, the predominant form of theanine found in tea, stimulates alpha brain waves that are associated with a relaxed but alert state of mind. Theanine may also help enhance your attention and focus. Because theanine helps the mind stop racing, it also seems to promote a more restful, sound sleep that is not interrupted by random thoughts.

But even teas without theanine can elevate GABA levels and promote relaxation. For optimal results, choose either a decaffeinated version of your favorite black or green tea or an herbal variety. Decaffeinated teas still have plenty of theanine. And while herbal teas are not really teas at all and do not contain theanine, these "tisanes," or herbal infusions made from the bark, leaves, and flowers of various plants, have plenty of other nutrients and health benefits.

The following herbal teas have specific GABA-enhancing properties.

Chamomile: A mild, relaxing tea with a delicate flavor, it contains oils that relax the smooth muscles in the stomach.

Lemon balm: Lemon balm reduces anxiety and restlessness, to tame tension and nervousness.

Passionflower: When sleep is disturbed by anxiety, passionflower is recommended.

PREGNENOLONE PUTS YOU IN THE MOOD

Pregnenolone is a naturally occurring hormone that is produced in the body from cholesterol. It is called the grandmother of hormones because the body uses it to create many other hormones, including testosterone, cortisone, progesterone, estrogen, DHEA, and others. Taking pregnenolone supplements allows you to keep all your hormones at more youthful levels. Pregnenolone also has a very calming effect: It appears to block the effects of cortisol release, preventing stress.

My patients often find that pregnenolone improves their energy, vision, memory, clarity of thinking, well-being, and often sexual enjoyment.

PROGESTERONE ENHANCES SEX BY FIXING YOUR MOOD

Progesterone is one of the "big three" sex hormones, along with estrogen and testosterone. Women produce progesterone in the ovaries, and men produce it in the adrenal glands. It is known to raise GABA levels, and in so doing acts as a natural antidepressant and tranquilizer. For the best results, you must take estrogen with progesterone, and progesterone with testosterone. In truth, you need all three for a balanced, natural approach to hormone replacement.

When progesterone levels drop, you can feel cranky or moody, both of which are not putting you in an ideal frame of mind for mind-blowing, orgasmic sex. Boosting levels of this hormone will help restore libido, improve mood, and enhance sleep patterns. Not only will you be able to have better sex, you'll sleep better, too.

Progesterone is prescribed to reduce libido in men with prostate problems and in

Relax on Your Own

People with a GABA SexQ desperately need time for themselves. Listening to music, reading quietly, taking solitary walks, exercising, or praying are all good ways to spend time without the rest of the world getting in the way. You may need to take an hour a day just to unwind. As your body adjusts to higher levels of GABA as well as more dopamine and acetylcholine, you may find you have less need to relax, but don't let go of this hour. Everyone deserves some time to do the things they enjoy. Once you have carved out this time, hold on to it.

violent criminals, including pedophiles and violent sex offenders. Women can use progesterone to slow down their sexuality, or to calm themselves down in general.

OXYTOCIN IMPROVES SEX BECAUSE IT PROMOTES BONDING

Oxytocin is the hormone directly linked with both male and female sexual response and is one of the most potent sexual stimulators because of its deep connection to human bonding. Oxytocin is related to GABA because it acts as a balancing, calming hormone. Released during any type of skin-to-skin contact, especially during sex, oxytocin makes us feel loved and secure, enhancing the sense of well-being. One interesting fact is that there are very few divorces in the first 3 months of a new baby's life, when oxytocin and bonding are plentiful.

Oxytocin causes contractions in the vagina, cervix, uterus, and penis by stimulating the smooth muscles of these organs. Oxytocin intensifies sexual receptivity by stimulating the body directly; in some ways, oxytocin circumvents an imbalanced brain. This is called reafference, meaning that initial physical stimulation leads to intensified nerve-genital-brain activity, which then causes an increased sensory response that intensifies the pleasurable feelings during orgasm.

Many sexual health experts believe, as I do, that if you supplement with oxytocin and stimulate these organs, both men and women can achieve increased and heightened orgasms, which is pivotal for younger, sexier sex. Women who are deficient in oxytocin may not be able to achieve orgasm at all and possibly have a weak desire for sex. Men who are deficient will lack the desire to be touched, as well as the ability to orgasm. Men who are high in dopamine and low in GABA may be able to use additional oxytocin to create better bonding with their partner. In return they will be less fooled by the conquest myth that casual intercourse can bring: that having sex with more women or younger women somehow enhances their value.

You can enhance your GABA production through hormones, foods, and nutrients, which will help maintain or enhance your levels of oxytocin. Or you can choose to work with your doctor to prescribe oxytocin supplements. Oxytocin supplementation has been common practice in hospital settings for dozens of years. Pitocin, the drug given to birthing mothers to increase contractions, is simply a synthetic form of oxytocin. However, prescribing a naturally compounded version that is more similar to the hormone we produce for increased sexual enjoyment is relatively new.

In my office, I have been treating men and women with natural, bioidentical oxytocin supplementation to improve their sex life. The feedback I've received is outstanding. Women experience deep vaginal contractions, and after a few weeks, many of my patients report that "sex felt the way it used to." These women also sense an increase in romantic attachment with their spouse and are able to form a closer, more connected relationship. I've had equally good results with my male patients: Oxytocin can restore ejaculation, increase sexual arousal, increase erection, and enhance orgasm.

This medication can be given as an injection or nasal spray, but I prefer a sublingual pill. It can be taken daily for a more consistent effect or before intercourse in larger doses. Dosages need to be addressed and adjusted for each patient, because an overload of oxytocin can have emotional and physical side effects. For example, it can lead to increased attachment anxiety, where people can become too clingy, too needy, especially when their partner isn't around.

TYPICAL OXYTOCIN DOSAGES

- Sublingual used for sexual arousal: 25–50 IU daily or 15 to 30 minutes before intercourse
- 40 units/ml nasal spray daily (1 spray)

Case Study: Olivia's Orgasms Were Weak

One of my favorite new patients is Olivia, a beautiful and vibrant 47-year-old who lives every day to its fullest. Olivia has a very important job as a human resources executive at a major international company, and her hectic work life had left little time for dating anyone too seriously. So when she met the man of her dreams at a business conference when she was 37, Olivia knew that the planets were aligned. She married Tom a year later, but the two of them were still too committed to their careers to think about children, until the unexpected happened. At 43, Olivia became a new mom.

Four years later, Olivia's sex life was like a dormant volcano: Nothing was happening, but she felt like she was going to explode from frustration. She was just too tired to have sex after working all day and taking care of her young daughter. Tom began to feel estranged from their relationship. Olivia was also upset that she couldn't lose her pregnancy weight. She knew that something had to change. She had just finished reading my book, *Younger (Thinner) You Diet,* and decided to fly in to see me.

Olivia's bloodwork showed that her hormone levels were very low. When she explained the kind of sexual relations she used to enjoy having, I realized immediately that she used to have a high dopamine SexQ, but her lack of dopamine had caused her metabolism to grind to a halt, and her fatigue was getting in the way of her sexual desire. I calmly explained that none of this was her fault. Her brain had just become chemically unbalanced, and her body was getting older than her actual age.

In just 1 month, I was able to teach Olivia how to rebalance her aging brain by improving her diet and increasing her hormone levels naturally. I prescribed progesterone and estrogen to rebalance her brain and started her on an oxytocin treatment to boost her sex drive. Olivia took the oxytocin daily as a sublingual tablet and almost immediately saw results. As she lost weight, her energy increased. And with the help of oxytocin, she was able to have great, passionate sex. Not only did her libido return, the intensity of her orgasms was heightened. In fact, Olivia told me that she was enjoying sex more now than she ever had before.

GABA MEDICATIONS MAKE YOU SEXUALLY CONFIDENT

GABA medications produce a mild feeling of euphoria and relieve anxiety. The following medications are currently prescribed to work with GABA to lessen anxiety and increase sexuality. Discuss them with your doctor to determine if they are necessary and if they will affect other health issues you may be experiencing.

- Xyrem may enhance female sexual desire by reducing sexual inhibitions. Also used to treat narcolepsy and daytime sleepiness.

- Carbamazepine, Carbatrol, Celontin, Dilantin, Epitol, Ethosuximide, Ethotoin, Felbamate, Felbatol, Fosphenytoin, Keppra, Lamictal, Lamotrigine, Levetiracetam, Mesantoin, Methsuximide, Milontin, Mysoline, Oxcarbazepine, Peganone, Phensuximide, Phenytoin, Primidone, Tegretol, Topamax, Topiramate, Tridione, Trileptal, Trimethadione, Zarontin, Zonegran, and Zonisamide are all mood stabilizers.
- BuSpar is an anxiety medication.
- Ativan, Dalmane, Diastat, Doral, Halcion, Klonopin, Librium, Paxipam, ProSom, Restoril, Serax, Tranxene-SD, Valium, and Xanax are all in the family of medications called benzodiazepines, which slow down the nervous system. Some are used to relieve anxiety; others to treat insomnia.

A CALM BRAIN = A BETTER SEX LIFE

The daily stresses of life can bring stress into the bedroom. Any suppressed emotions, including anger, resentment, hostility, heartbreak, even sadness, are signs that

Ancient Chinese Secret

According to the tenets of Chinese medicine, sexual activity unleashes an exchange of energy between the yang (sun/man) and yin (earth/woman). Energy particles from the sun continually enter the fingers, travel through the arms and rest of the body, and pass through the toes, while energy from the earth travels in the opposite direction. Illness is said to occur if there is an imbalance in this system, and the act of sex is noted for its ability to increase the flow of this energy, promoting health and longevity.

something is not right in your life. But your SexQ will determine how you handle life's stresses. For those with a GABA-dominant brain, all this pent-up stress may eventually make you sick, or worse.

Sex is the ideal way to relieve stress. Even if you can't confront the source of your stress, a good session in bed with your partner can go a long way toward releasing the tension. And if you choose to deal with your personal issues in a therapeutic way, you can still have sex. Of course, exercise also relieves stress, but good sex is better for your relationship than a good run.

CHAPTER 7

Serotonin Keeps the Joy in Sex

THE SEROTONIN SexQ is interested in sex and regards it as a recreational sport. Serotonin is the brain chemical that allows you to experience pleasure and feel good about yourself, so when you have plenty of it, you are able to live in the moment and experience sex as just plain fun.

If you scored high in the serotonin section of the quiz in Chapter 3, you might be more likely to think of sex as a game in which you can keep score. You remember your best orgasm and measure each subsequent one against it, because you are so impressed by what you've done—and what you know you're capable of. Sexual performance is important to you and a part of what defines you: You know how many partners you have had and what each of them did for you. When you are in a relationship, you feel deeply about your spouse/partner, and when you are not, the world is like one big love-in, and you are willing to share yourself with anyone.

When your serotonin levels are high, you feel alive and vibrant during the day. At night, serotonin allows you to experience deep, restful sleep so the brain can recharge, and every morning is a fresh start. When your brain is balanced and refreshed, it's a whole lot easier to have sex. In fact, just getting plenty of restful sleep will give you 10 more years of great sex.

TOO MUCH SEROTONIN LEAVES YOU UNSATISFIED

So far I've discussed the upside of strong serotonin levels in the brain. Like anything, though, you can have too much of a good thing. When you have too much serotonin, sex isn't just a game, it's an obsession. A person with a high serotonin SexQ is a thrill seeker who may be willing to try almost anything to achieve the best orgasm ever—or even just another one. Yet high serotonin brain sex can get funky very quickly, as you progress from trying new sexual positions to having sex in more challenging ways or with multiple partners. Think of being stuck in the 1970s at Plato's Retreat, all day, every day.

While taking this walk on the wild side may sound exciting, you run the risk of relinquishing a more balanced way of living. You wind up stuck in the adolescence of sex, never capable of growing up and committing to a deeply loving relationship. In order to achieve more balance, not only will you have to balance your brain chemicals, but you'll also need to channel some of that thrill-seeking into your daily life and out of your bedroom so that you can have more meaningful, more intimately connected sex.

Your fixation on sexual adventure may be just one symptom of a brain chemical imbalance. With too much serotonin, your timing is off, which for men can mean premature ejaculation (PE). High-serotonin men can even experience orgasm without erection.

While calling an ejaculation premature is to some degree subjective (whose expectation is it anyway, and who's to say how long sex should last?), it is usually defined as the tendency to ejaculate appreciably more quickly than would be required for a man's own satisfaction or that of his partner. Typically, unwanted ejaculation occurs within the first minute of intercourse and may even occur before penetration. You'll learn more about PE and erectile dysfunction (ED) in Chapters 9 and 10, but for now it's important to recognize their connection to levels of serotonin in the brain. However, problems with high serotonin are not exclusive to men: Women with too

Can You Ever Have Too Much Fun?

According to a 2004 ABC News poll, 16 percent of US adults admitted to having had an affair. If you fall into this category, you may need to dial down your playful "no commitments" serotonin nature and balance your SexQ by enhancing the other brain chemicals. More dopamine will give your sex life more focus. More acetylcholine may let you see your current lover in a more romantic light. More GABA will give you a renewed sense of confidence in your relationship so that you'll stop playing the field.

much serotonin can experience prolonged delays in orgasm, which includes the need for extended stimulation in order to achieve orgasm.

LOVE IS . . . AN EXERCISE IN BRAIN CHEMISTRY

Romantic love is characterized by a euphoric feeling when things are going well, and terrible mood swings when they're not. Now that you understand brain chemistry, you can see that your love life is connected directly to the brain.

Helen Fisher, PhD, of Rutgers University, used functional magnetic resonance imagery (fMRI) to create a scientific scenario showing that romantic love is not an emotional reaction at all. Rather, it's the way the brain rewards us (dopamine!) for finding an appropriate mating partner. We also know that when dopamine is high, serotonin is often low. Low serotonin allows you to be more vulnerable so that you can fall in love. It forces the brain toward

Not All Antidepressants Are Great for Sex

People who have too much serotonin are often taking antidepressants. While these drugs may alleviate the symptoms of depression and allow you to get restful sleep, they make it very difficult to achieve orgasm. Selective serotonin reuptake inhibitors (SSRIs) are known to inhibit orgasm, while tricyclic antidepressants (TCAs) are more likely to cause erectile dysfunction. You should never be embarrassed to talk about these types of side effects with your doctor, who can make changes in your medication so that your mood, as well as your sex life, won't suffer.

focused attention, obsessive thinking, and intense cravings for that special someone. Once the bond is set and the reward is met, dopamine drops and serotonin rises. That's when the fun starts: Dating and early stages of relationships mean lots of fun sex, lots of good times. Eventually, though, both you and your relationship mature. The dopamine brain doesn't have to be so powerful because it has already received its mating reward. And the serotonin brain becomes more stable. In the best-case scenario, your loving brain becomes balanced, and so does your sex life. In the worst case, low dopamine means no sexual desire, and low serotonin jeopardizes the connection between your feelings and reality.

TOO LITTLE SEROTONIN MAKES YOU UNHAPPY

Hypogonadism occurs in men and women when the sex glands produce little or no hormones. While we've already shown how this can affect your sex life, it can also induce depression. Bioidentical hormone replacement therapies can restore hormones to more youthful levels, reversing sexual dysfunction and improving mood.

When your serotonin levels begin to wane, you may notice your moods changing for the worse. While dopamine and GABA deficiencies affect your emotional life, and acetylcholine affects your intellectual life, serotonin deficiencies are markedly different—and even more pronounced. Instead of feeling fatigued (low dopamine), slow-witted (acetylcholine), or anxious (low GABA), without serotonin you don't feel much of anything, including sexual desire. When you try to perk yourself up, you may find that your sex life has suddenly become out of sync. Many people who have a serotonin deficiency are trapped in a cycle of obsessive thinking about romantic love. In another study by Dr. Fisher, depressed individuals were shown to spend as much as 95 percent of their day thinking about their loved one.

Another common trait among those deficient in serotonin is a perception of themselves as outlaws or rule breakers. They become overly impulsive and shortsighted, stomping through life without considering consequences. They have sex with whomever they want, whenever they want.

The physical symptoms of low serotonin can cause an emotional response, and vice versa. Painful orgasms or pains during sexual activity are common symptoms. Men may

Serotonin Sexual Archetypes

Too Much: Wilt Chamberlain—this former basketball star never married and admitted in his autobiography that he had slept with 20,000 women

Too Little: Marilyn Monroe—in the end she was haunted by depression and failed marriages

require more stimulation than usual to maintain an erection and may have difficulty maintaining an erection long enough to complete the sex act. Low serotonin skin is literally numb: The nipples, clitoris, and genitals lack sensation.

Both men and women can become depressed when their sex lives wither, and conversely depression itself can cause them to lose interest in sex. In my practice I've found that more than 50 percent of patients who suffer from erectile dysfunction also suffer from depression.

A mild depression may last for only a day or two, but a major depression can last many months or years. Some people, particularly men, experience mild depression following sex—even great sex—that can last up to a day. This phenomenon is called postcoital tristesse, or "sadness after sex."

And here's the worst part: When it comes to depression, the treatment may cause further sexual dysfunction. As I noted earlier, one common source of low libido and changes in sexual performance is the use of antidepressants known as selective serotonin reuptake inhibitors (SSRIs), including Prozac and Zoloft. These medications often create a drop in sex drive or anorgasmia, meaning desire is there but you can't orgasm. Some antidepressants are also linked to reduced clitoral sensation in women and inability to achieve erection and smaller quantities of seminal fluid in men. SSRIs flood the bloodstream with serotonin, lowering the need for the brain to create its own. Because SSRIs raise serotonin without increasing dopamine, those who take it feel good about themselves without feeling the need to seek sexual reward. SSRIs also muffle emotions, including the elation of romance, and suppress obsessive thinking, a critical component to falling in love.

Fortunately, researchers are working on antidepressants that can also increase dopamine. Bupropion, for example, enhances the brain's production of dopamine and may be a substitute for SSRIs.

SIGNS OF A LOW SEROTONIN SexQ:

- I'm too sad to have sex.
- I'm easily irritated.
- I crave carbohydrates and salty snacks.
- I've had self-destructive or suicidal thoughts.
- I frequently take sleeping pills.

YOU NEED SLEEP FOR BETTER SEX

As you age, the quality of your rest deteriorates, even if you are getting the same number of hours of shut-eye. When your serotonin levels fall, you don't get as much REM (rapid eye movement) sleep, the deepest, most restorative sleep phase. Too little REM sleep is one of the great age accelerators, prematurely aging your brain, your body, and your sex life. Poor sleep does not allow the brain to reboot overnight to get ready for the next day. A lack of sleep can exacerbate any disease, triggering inflammation. And, when you do not achieve a deep sleep state, all your fears, phobias, obsessions, compulsions, and blues become exaggerated, resulting in a continuous loop of mental symptoms that feed physical ones and negatively impact your sex drive and performance.

A surprisingly large number of people have reported participating in sexual activity during sleep. In a 2010 study from the Sleep and Alertness Clinic at University Health Network's Toronto Western Hospital, 7.6 percent of participants reported either having had sex or engaging in other sexual activity, like masturbation, while asleep. While this sounds fun, it's not. The author of the study, Dr. Sharon A. Chung, reminds us that any disruption of the sleep cycle is a problem, not an opportunity.

If you have a serotonin deficiency, your brain's delta waves are actually more elevated during the day, blocking alertness (dopamine), creativity (acetylcholine), and playfulness (GABA). At night, poor sleep can manifest itself in different ways. You may have difficulty falling asleep, and you may wake in the middle of the night and be unable to go back to sleep. You might be plagued with night terrors or nightmares, wake up frequently to go to the bathroom, or never get to sleep at all, tossing and worrying all night long.

Better sleep helps sex, and many GABA agents make sleep more possible. For example, a GABA medication, Rohypnol (flunitrazepam), is known as the date-rape drug, because as a heavy tranquilizer it suppresses will, or allows people to let go of their will, which proves exactly how brain chemistry can alter sexuality and sexual choice.

Sex Might Only Take 15 Minutes, But You Need 7 Hours of Sleep

That's your goal. Here are some easy tips to help you get there.

- Try to go to bed at the same time each night.
- Set up a nighttime routine that does not involve television or working on the computer immediately before bed. Instead,

Morning Missiles Show Men That They're Getting Good Sleep

Outside of a scientific sleep study, the only way to know if you are getting enough sleep is to consider how you feel in the morning—and I mean how you feel *everywhere*. For men, waking up with an erection is a sure sign that the brain is balanced. These morning missiles prove that your body and brain are ready for younger sex. Just make sure that your partner had a good night's sleep as well.

listen to some sexy, relaxing music in a darkened bedroom.

- Don't eat for at least 3 hours before you go to bed.
- Sleep in a cool, dark room that is only used for "bedroom" activities. Make sure that air flow and ventilation are good.
- Lavender-scented candles, aromatherapy oil, or night cream relaxes the mind before bed.
- Do not have coffee, alcohol, or cigarettes before bed (no cigarettes, ever!).
- Don't fall asleep on the couch: Get into bed the moment you realize you are sleepy.
- Avoid naps in the late afternoon or early evening.
- Take serotonin-enhancing supplements 1 hour before you plan to go to sleep.

Case Study: Catherine Couldn't Climax

When Catherine came to see me last year, she was both agitated and excited. At 77, she had a long history of depression and high cholesterol, and had significant weight gain around her midsection. She had lost her husband 10 years earlier and hadn't thought about sex much since. But recently she had met a man in a dance class at her local senior center, and they had started dating. Within a few months she was engaged. The only problem was that she was troubled by her lack of interest in sex, even though she felt deeply in love and profoundly connected to her fiancé. The truth was that Catherine had never had an orgasm during her first marriage and was afraid of disappointing her new husband.

I told Catherine that an active sex life was not only possible, but necessary for her long-term health. I explained that it is never too late to enhance a SexQ, and a new marriage affords a great opportunity to create a new beginning.

I administered my SexQ quiz, as well as a complete physical, so we could rule out underlying issues that might be affecting her sexuality. I found that Catherine was in relatively good health overall, but the quiz suggested that she had a serotonin SexQ. I suggested that she stop taking her antidepressants, which might have been contributing to her inability to orgasm or her decreased desire for sex. Instead, I prescribed a bioidentical hormone regimen that would help her feel younger. It included estradiol, progesterone, topical testosterone cream, DHEA supplements, pregnenolone, growth hormone, and thyroid hormone. At first Catherine was overwhelmed by the sheer number of medications that I prescribed, since she believed that menopause was 20 years behind her. However, I explained that menopause is not a onetime event but an ongoing condition, and that by enhancing her natural hormone levels, she would not only feel younger, but she would feel sexier.

Within 3 months, Catherine's life changed completely. Her depression and anxiety lifted. She was able to lose weight and had more energy for planning her wedding. Best of all, she found that her sexual desire was strong, and on her wedding night she achieved an orgasm for the first time in her life. Catherine now feels a greater sense of confidence than ever before, and regrets only that she did not start this therapy sooner!

SEX UP YOUR SEROTONIN BY EATING FOODS HIGH IN TRYPTOPHAN

Tryptophan is an amino acid that the brain and body need but cannot make on their own. It is vital for those with low serotonin because it induces the creation of this brain chemical. Tryptophan is so effective in creating more serotonin that you might see your moods improve soon after eating foods that contain it in abundance. For example, if you feel sad, eating tryptophan-rich foods can quickly improve your mood and even increase your libido.

If you are low in serotonin, you should have at least 2 grams of tryptophan every day. Choose from the foods listed below.

Foods High in Tryptophan

FOOD	GRAMS OF TRYPTOPHAN PER 6–8 OZ SERVING
Pork	1.00
Avocado	0.40
Cottage cheese	0.40
Duck	0.40
Eggs	0.40
Wheat germ	0.40
Turkey	0.37
Chicken	0.28
Chocolate	0.11

Foods to Choose When You're Feeling Blue

One Finnish study found that people who frequently eat fish with high concentrations of omega-3 fatty acids, such as salmon, are 31 percent less likely to suffer from depression. Besides salmon, other fish that can improve your mood are trout, herring, sardines, and mackerel. These choices are high in vitamin B_{12}, a GABA nutrient that can also be found in eggs, sea vegetables, soybean products, and kelp and can provide a similar feeling of calmness as other serotonin agents.

Aside from fish, other good choices for boosting serotonin are foods packed with the nutrient biotin, including egg yolks, soybeans, and whole grains; or foods high in purine, such as calf's liver and flat mushrooms. High-purine foods should be avoided if you have gout.

Use Spices to Perk Yourself Up

Many spices have antidepressant properties, naturally increasing your serotonin levels. Saffron, for example, is clinically shown to help depression and doesn't have the sexual side effects often associated with medications like Prozac and Imipramine. Other good choices include marjoram, peppermint, spearmint, and dill.

Nutmeg, licorice (anise), and turmeric have scientifically proven potent antidepressant activity. In a 2006 experiment using mice, nutmeg extract was shown to be comparable to the prescription medicines Imipramine and Fluoxetine in several standard tests. Specifically, nutmeg was shown to markedly affect levels of adrenaline, dopamine, and serotonin. One theory is that the active compounds in nutmeg have pharmacological properties similar to amphetamines and the recreational drug Ecstasy. The same year, an Indian study achieved similar results with licorice. A 2002 study of turmeric from Nanjing University in Jiangsu, China, also showed a correlation between the spice and MAO inhibition.

CREATE MORE SEROTONIN FOR MORE JOYFUL SEX

Another way to increase tryptophan and other serotonin-boosting nutrients is through vitamin and mineral supplements. The following nutrients will help relax your brain so you feel less depressed and more confident, which is integral to having better sex.

Most should be taken in the late evening because they will make you drowsy. Please note that these supplements may interfere with your medications, especially if you are already taking antidepressants, so it is essential that you consult your health care provider to see which of the following may be appropriate for you.

TREATMENT	SUGGESTED DAILY DOSAGE	HOW IT AFFECTS SEX
Magnesium	200–500 mg	May help with premature ejaculation.
Melatonin	0.5–3 mg	In animal research (rats), small amounts of melatonin caused males to have sex more rapidly and frequently. Melatonin may also increase blood flow to the penis.
SAMe	400–1,600 mg	Taken in the morning, SAMe may help with depression and also contributes to the activation of several brain chemicals and hormones. A form of methionine, it's often used to treat fatty liver, arthritis, and depression.
St. John's wort	500–1,000 mg (std. to hypericin or hyperforin)	May be as effective for depression as many prescription medications. Helps to resolve premature ejaculations, social phobias, avoidance, and dysthymia (the blues).
Tryptophan	500–2,000 mg	Can increase the effectiveness of prescription antidepressants and provides additional serotonin. Helps to resolve premature ejaculation, sleep disorders, insomnia, shortened sleep cycle, and dependency on SSRIs.
Vitamin D	1,000–5,000 IU	Elevates mood. May help with depression and seasonal affective disorder (SAD) and heart disease.

SEROTONIN-ENHANCING MEDICATIONS

Sexual difficulties were at one time thought to be almost exclusively psychological in origin. Today we know that for as many as 50 percent of men suffering from erectile dysfunction, a biological cause may be at least partly to blame. In such cases, taking action will mean taking medicine.

Prescribing a serotonin medication alone may not address the whole issue, especially because so many serotonin agents will compromise your sex life. For example, in a study completed at the University of California, San Francisco, researchers conclusively found that antidepressant-induced sexual dysfunction (ASD) resulted in testosterone levels that were below the normal ranges for 75 percent of both men and women.

However, serotonin medications combined with bioidentical hormones, nutrients, and lifestyle changes provide the greatest benefits. When a woman can't have an orgasm, she needs to increase serotonin. When a man suffers from premature ejacu-lation, he needs to decrease serotonin. Some antidepressants like Paxil or Prozac can enhance sexual satisfaction by slowing down your sexual response.

Antidepressant Drugs That Treat Sexual Disorders

GENERIC NAME	BRAND NAME	HOW IT AFFECTS SEX
Amitriptyline	Elavil	Diminishes premature ejaculation by decreasing serotonin
Bupropion	Wellbutrin	Increases ability to orgasm by increasing serotonin
Buspirone	BuSpar	Increases ability to orgasm by increasing serotonin
Citalopram	Celexa	Diminishes premature ejaculation by decreasing serotonin
Clomipramine	Anafranil	Diminishes premature ejaculation by decreasing serotonin
Desipramine	Norpramin	Diminishes premature ejaculation by decreasing serotonin
Duloxetine	Cymbalta	Increases ability to orgasm by increasing serotonin
Escitalopram oxalate	Lexapro	Diminishes premature ejaculation by decreasing serotonin
Fluoxetine	Prozac	Diminishes premature ejaculation by decreasing serotonin
Fluvoxamine	Luvox	Diminishes premature ejaculation by decreasing serotonin
Imipramine	Tofranil	Diminishes premature ejaculation by decreasing serotonin
Mirtazapine	Remeron	Increases ability to orgasm by increasing serotonin
Moclobemide	Aurorix	Increases ability to orgasm by increasing serotonin
Nortriptyline	Pamelor	Diminishes premature ejaculation by decreasing serotonin
Paroxetine	Paxil	Diminishes premature ejaculation by decreasing serotonin
Reboxetine	Edronax	Increases ability to orgasm by increasing serotonin
Sertraline	Zoloft	Diminishes premature ejaculation by decreasing serotonin
Trazodone	Desyrel	Increases ability to orgasm by increasing serotonin
Venlafaxine	Effexor	Diminishes premature ejaculation by decreasing serotonin

Serotonin Medications Especially for Men

- Bethanechol: may increase sexual desire in men whose sexual desire is impaired resulting from excessive use of antidepressants
- Muse (Alprostadil Penile Suppository): used as needed to achieve an erection; the effect starts about 5 minutes after application and lasts about 30 to 60 minutes
- Viagra, Levitra, Cialis: can prevent ED (see Chapter 10)

THE BALANCED SEXUAL ADVANTAGE

The optimum SexQ is one where all the brain chemicals are balanced. But a balanced SexQ takes time and commitment. I have seen amazing results from my patients who follow my protocol based on their unique brain chemistry. I know that if you stick with this, you will, too.

Without sex, the brain atrophies. But when your brain chemistry is perfectly balanced, you'll be able to achieve what I call a *full brain orgasm*. Not only will you feel a more passionate, intense orgasm, you'll experience the sensation of total happiness combined with cognitive enhancement, followed by deep, relaxing sleep. This occurs because all four brain chemicals are being simultaneously released in the right proportions.

The rest of the book more closely examines how hormonal loss affects your SexQ, and your overall health. You'll learn new ways to improve your health so that you can capture and maintain your balanced SexQ for years to come.

PART II

Younger (Sexier) You for Women

CHAPTER 8

Beat Menopause and Perimenopause to Enhance Your SexQ

WHEN IT COMES to aging, there are two undeniable facts every woman should know. First, men and women age differently in every conceivable way. And second, menopause starts earlier than you think. Once you come to terms with this, you'll be able to comprehend everything you need to know in order to feel younger and sexier for years to come. And, you'll finally understand why men and women behave so differently when it comes to sex.

The gender differences that govern your health begin in the brain: They are not limited to your reproductive organs. In utero, your brain is programmed as definitively male or female, releasing different amounts of brain chemicals that govern hormone levels accordingly. Extra estrogen hits the brain of a baby girl; extra testosterone hits the brain of a baby boy. No matter what you do to the outside of your body, and to some extent, how you treat your insides, you will always be gender-rigged as inherently male or female.

Because men and women are different, their sexuality ages at different rates. Men can maintain their sexuality longer than women. That's not a theory, that's a fact. Men lose testosterone and other hormones at a much slower rate, and they do so later in life than women, which means that they are ready, willing, and able to have sex for most of their adult lives. However, women's hormone levels start to drop almost from the moment they enter adulthood, which means that just when they master the pleasures of sex, they are genetically programmed to desire it less and less.

Hard as it may be to accept, perimenopause begins as early as 22. By the age of 30, women experience a change in their hormones and temporarily experience a more active sexual period. However, by the age of 40, the brain becomes less effective at sending messages to the other organs that produce hormones, which forces the organs to age. Hormone levels decline as you age. By the time you reach your forties and fifties, if you are not paying attention to your fitness and your health, your declining hormones will bring your sex life crashing down and your health along with it. The number one thing that you can do to enhance and keep your sex life active is to treat menopause early.

I reverse my female patients' symptoms of menopause every single day, and in the process restore their sexuality. These treatments help my patients lose weight, increase muscle mass, increase libido, increase arousal, increase their ability to achieve orgasm, and get rid of their depression. They go from wanting to have sex once a month to looking forward to having sex three times a week or more. As they achieve sexual parity with their spouse or partner, their health and mental well-being bloom as well.

HORMONES ARE NOTHING TO BE AFRAID OF

Hormones are chemicals produced by glands, and there are more than 100 different hormones in a healthy body. The brain regulates, translates, and interprets its electrical code as hormonal output from the various internal organs. When hormone output is high, you feel healthy, sexy, and young.

As women age, internal organs get to a point where they fail to produce their related hormones on their own. Without natural hormone supplementation, that organ will die and drag your overall health down with it. The brain tries desperately to resurrect the dying organ by sending additional electrical signals to the hypothalamus, which in turn begins to release hormones to the pituitary gland. This action stimulates the ovaries, adrenal glands, thyroid, or liver in an attempt to reverse the aging process. But no such luck. Instead, the body releases excess cortisol, and we end up feeling anxious and collecting belly fat.

Meanwhile, despite your best efforts to counteract the combined effects of gravity and aging, your arms, legs, and torso have probably been getting progressively flabbier since the age of 30: The typical woman begins losing muscle mass starting around 25, as hormone levels begin to decline.

Hormones like estrogen, progesterone, testosterone, pregnenolone, androstenedione, and dehydroepiandrosterone (DHEA) all derive from cholesterol, a waxy, fatlike substance that is necessary for your overall health. Cholesterol is an essential component of every cell and is required by the body to perform certain functions: It

Aging Is a Giant Neuropathy

The whole body grows numb with age, and we lose that exquisite, incredible skin sensitivity of youth. The only way to turn a prune back into a plum is with a total antiaging, sex-enhancing program that balances brain chemistry while restoring more youthful levels of hormones. What's more, the right diet, including nutritional supplements, provides the daily balance women need to keep their metabolisms high so that they can physically look and feel younger and sexier.

lubricates the body, helping the blood flow smoothly. It is usually produced in the liver, but if the body requires more than the liver can produce, it will create its own cholesterol from the foods we eat. However, if too much cholesterol is produced, it begins to collect inside the walls of blood vessels. When this happens, cholesterol turns from a helpful necessity to a harmful substance. Cholesterol levels naturally rise as we age, but eventually the ovaries and adrenal glands cannot keep up with the job of converting cholesterol into hormones. The result is reduced hormone levels accompanied by reduced sexual motivation and function, both of which are total body symptoms of hormone deficiency.

For many women, perimenopause can look and feel as much like a march into "shrinkhood" as menopause itself: They lose height, get weaker, notice dry and wrinkled skin as well as decreased sensitivity to touch, and end up seeking the advice of a real shrink because they think they're going crazy. Symptoms and their severity vary from woman to woman; some experience almost none, while others may experience any combination of the following:

- Aching joints
- Attention deficiencies
- Backache
- Bladder infection
- Breast tenderness
- Cold sweats
- Confusion
- Constipation
- Decreased bone density
- Depression
- Diarrhea
- Dizzy spells
- Dry eyes
- Dry nose and mouth
- Dry skin
- Facial hair growth
- Fatigue
- Fine lines around mouth and eyes
- Headaches
- Hot flashes
- Increased gas
- Increased incidence of cysts
- Insomnia
- Irritability
- Irritable bowel syndrome
- Lack of energy
- Loss of appetite
- Memory loss
- Mood swings
- Nervous tension
- Night sweats
- Persistent cough
- Rapid heartbeat
- Shortness of breath
- Skin rash/irritation
- Sore throat
- Swelling
- Thinning hair or hair loss
- Tingling in hands and feet
- Urinary incontinence, discomfort, or changes in frequency
- Vaginal discharge
- Vaginal dryness

If You See Something, Say Something

A diminished sex life does not have to be just another accepted part of aging, and you're not doing yourself a favor by keeping sexual discomfort a secret. This isn't something you have to live with, and it might be a signal that there is a bigger health problem lurking somewhere. But most important, remember that sex affects every aspect of the quality of your life, and any discomfort can be treated. Don't be embarrassed to talk to your doctor about sex. The first step is to bring a list of your symptoms to your doctor. Together, you'll come up with a plan that can restore your sexuality and improve your quality of life.

- Vaginal numbness
- Weakness
- Weight gain

THE DIFFERENCE BETWEEN PERIMENOPAUSE AND MENOPAUSE

Menopause is often referred to as the change, but this term is misleading. It implies that the changes associated with menopause are a onetime occurrence. Unfortunately, this is not the case. Women begin perimenopause as early as 10 to 15 years before full menopause hits. During perimenopause, your ovaries continue to release eggs, and you will continue to ovulate and menstruate. Once you have begun menopause, ovulation completely stops. And just as the changes associated with perimenopause occur gradually, the seemingly abrupt changes of menopause actually continue for many years after ovulation ends.

Many factors influence the age at which you begin perimenopause, including:

- Family genetics
- Depression
- Exposure to environmental toxins such as smoking, chemotherapy, irradiation
- Obesity
- Prior oral contraceptive use
- Stress

During the transition from perimenopause to menopause, your menstrual flow can change erratically, which can impact your sex life. Expect any of the following:

- Heavy periods accompanied by blood clots
- Periods that last several days longer than usual
- Spotting between periods
- Spotting after sex
- Periods that occur closer together
- Light periods
- Skipped periods

You can also expect changes in your sex drive. For example, Meg was just 44 when she told me about her severely decreased libido. Her blood work showed that her hormonal balances were completely off-kilter, even though she was still getting her period. I started Meg on a few bioidentical hormonal supplements, which worked quickly and effectively. Natural estrogen, progesterone, and testosterone helped Meg boost her libido, and she was soon back to feeling sexy!

THE STAGES OF MENOPAUSE

For women ages 22 to 40, two naturally occurring hormones are poised to kill your sex life: leuteinizing hormone (LH) and follicle-stimulating hormone (FSH). Women who take—or have taken—birth control pills may have an artificially lower baseline number than women who haven't, yet as we age and these hormones increase, they can damage your brain and consequently affect your desire for sex. The stages of menopause are determined by an increase in production of FSH, so be sure to have your blood levels tested for these numbers every year starting at age 30.

Stage 1: Premenopause/late reproductive stage: Begins while you are still fertile, so there is a healthy quality and quantity of egg cells in the ovaries. At this point there is a minimal increase in FSH.

Stage 2: Perimenopause: FSH levels increase in comparison to baseline levels. This is accompanied by a decline in quantity and quality of egg cells, and your ability to become pregnant diminishes.

Stage 3: Late perimenopause: Significant increases of FSH; infrequent occurrence of menstrual cycle.

Stage 4: Menopause: High FSH levels plateau; complete cessation of menstrual cycle.

The symptoms of perimenopause and menopause can be surprising and often upsetting, and without properly addressing them there will be times when you think that you are truly losing your mind.

Forgetfulness, erratic behavior, and dramatic moodiness are just some of the symptoms that cause women to think they are losing emotional control. The reality is that if we can replace hormones to the level of a 23-year-old in a 35-year-old woman, she'll be a better lover than she was when she was 22, because she will have the wisdom of age plus the desire of youth. What's more, she won't be plagued by poor emotional control and will be better able to handle the stresses of marriage and life.

With more youthful hormone levels, you can achieve better marital bonding. But you have to want it and be ready for it. I've seen women who are so filled with resentment toward their spouse that they don't *want* to bond. They may feel excluded by the connection between their children and their husband. So many different things affect a mature marriage that people become comfortable in their unhappiness and fear change. I firmly believe that change is almost always for the better.

However, if you are ready to rewind your hormonal clock 15, 20, or even 30 years, then you have to expect, and watch out for, a new level of personal volatility. You can have the more aggressive and assertive dopamine libido. You can become the romantic acetylcholine woman who is excited by the touch of her partner. But you have to learn how to stabilize that revitalized sexual energy with some GABA.

Menopause Doesn't Have to Affect Sex

The only way you can stay sexually vibrant is to keep your hormone levels high and stay physically fit and healthy. If you enhance your brain chemistry as soon as you experience the slightest changes in your sex life, you will be able to remain younger and sexier. If you are a woman between the ages of 35 and 45, now is the perfect time to combat the effects of menopause with an antiaging program before the symptoms damage your overall quality of life. And if you are older and have already experienced the symptoms of menopause, you can reverse them simply by following my brain-balancing program.

Correcting hormone imbalances completely rejuvenates the body and the brain. There is no better way to make yourself feel younger than to be able to enjoy frequent, long-lasting sex. This will also have a welcome spin-off effect, not just in heightened sexual desire and performance, but in improvements of all health-related aspects of your life, since sexuality is a marker of overall health.

Replacing Lost Hormones Is Worth 15 More Years of Good Sex

It is so surprising to me that conventional medicine still doesn't get what's best for women. Doctors generally do little to help women who are suffering from symptoms of hormonal change. Even today, menopausal women are frequently sent home with a prescription for antidepressants rather than being offered real solutions for a very real condition. Antidepressants are not a *wrong* treatment for hot flashes; they're just incomplete.

Menopause is a natural stage of life that every woman must face. But that doesn't mean you have to suffer. In fact, menopause might herald the best years of your life.

My motto is to treat women as early as possible so that they never have to experience cognitive decline, flabbiness, muscle loss, and changes to their sexuality. Without an anti-aging program, the average 30-year-old woman is setting herself up to miss out on the joys of the later years of life. Remember, aging is inevitable. However, you can choose how you will age.

The best prescription for menopause is to naturally replace all the hormones that your body is no longer making, or making at less than optimal levels. In doing so, you are virtually turning back time to the health you enjoyed at 40, which is optimal for younger sex. If you want a more active sex life, you can ratchet up your SexQ even further, to regain the sexual interest of a 20- to 30-year-old.

Many hormones are precursors to, or act just like, specific brain chemicals. Replacing these missing hormones can boost your sex drive as well as your metabolism (by increasing dopamine), increase your ability

Great Advice for Great Sex

Following the Younger (Sexier) You program, which focuses on nutrients, herbs, spices, and teas, is essential for women between 30 and 50. Nutrients that enhance dopamine keep your sexual desire strong. Foods that increase acetylcholine will keep your mind sharp and at the same time strengthen your bones to prevent osteoporosis. Teas and herbs that increase GABA and serotonin keep your brain calm and relaxed.

to become aroused as well as reinvigorate your mental awareness (by increasing acetylcholine), increase your ability to experience orgasms and decrease anxiety (by increasing GABA), and allow you to get better sleep after loving, intimate sex (by increasing serotonin). By addressing these four aspects of your sexual well-being as well as the age accelerators, you will extend your sexual time line: With a healthy brain and a healthy body you'll be able to engage in comfortable, orgasmic, loving sex well into old age.

THE BEST SEX REQUIRES NATURAL BIOIDENTICAL HORMONES

Another fact: All hormone therapies are not created equal. In 2002, an enormous federally financed study was released from the Women's Health Initiative. With more than 10 years of research and 16,000 participants, the study found that hormone replacement therapy was dangerous. The women on hormones were having more heart trouble and their risk for stroke and blood clots increased, as did their risk for breast cancer. Synthetic estrogen and progesterone have also been linked to weight gain. Growth

hormone from cadavers has also been shown to cause cancer.

When the findings were released, many women quickly stopped taking their HRTs, and for good reason. What the media didn't pick up on was that the hormones in the study were completely synthetic, derived from horse urine. I've been saying for more than a decade that synthetic hormones are dangerous: Now science was on my side. Yet to this day, they are being prescribed by doctors across the country. Some women have been prescribed birth control pills to ease perimenopausal or menopausal symptoms, but I don't recommend this because the Pill can ruin your mood, your libido, your sleep, and your health.

I prescribe only bioidentical hormones, which are plant-based, natural, and safe. These compounds have the exact same molecular structure as those produced by the human body, and therefore they produce the same physiologic responses as the body's natural hormones. Bioidentical hormones have been available for more than 20 years and cause so few side effects that many are sold over the counter as nutrient supplements (melatonin, pregnenolone, vitamin D_3, and DHEA to name a few). They are an effective way to alleviate symptoms of menopause and perimenopause without adding dangerous, synthetic toxins to your already taxed body. At the same time, these bioidentical hormones will jump-start your brain's chemical production, especially of dopamine and acetylcholine, which is exactly what you need to enhance your sex drive.

There is a wide range of hormones that you can consider replacing with bioidenticals, depending on your current health status. Often a combination is most effective. For example, virtually all women need to take estrogen, progesterone, and testosterone to maintain the right blood level of estrogen, even if they are only experiencing symptoms related to one issue. Read through the following list carefully, and discuss with your doctor which of these choices is right for you.

The Best of the Bioidenticals

Calcitonin is produced by the thyroid gland and affects bone growth and calcium regulation. It is generally administered as a nasal spray or through injection. It can be obtained with a doctor's prescription and is usually prescribed for women experiencing the earliest stages of loss of bone density.

DHEA is produced in the adrenal cortex and in the brain. It is then converted to estrogen and testosterone. DHEA is the main hormone that affects female libido. It can also facilitate weight loss as it works as a dopamine agent. Reestablishing DHEA balance

to original youthful levels can enhance sexual desire, receptivity, and performance, and restore the pleasure derived from sex. It is also used for chronic fatigue syndrome, depression, memory loss, menopause, osteoporosis, and to protect the body from the ravages of age. It can be purchased over the counter as a supplement. Watch for products with labels indicating they contain "7 Keto DHEA." This formulation does not convert or metabolize into testosterone and estradiol in the same way as DHEA. However, there are many studies that show it improves the immune system and cuts down on gut fat.

Erythropoietin (EPO) is produced by the kidneys and is the hormone that regulates red blood cell production in the bone marrow. It is used to treat anemia and has been studied for its ability to improve libido. It can also be used as a way to improve sexual functioning for women who suffer from scleroderma, a condition of extremely tight, hard skin. This bioidentical hormone can be obtained with a doctor's prescription.

Estradiol (E2) is a sex hormone produced by the ovaries and the adrenal cortex. It is the predominant sex hormone present in premenopausal women, and through supplementation may increase sexual desire by stimulating the production of nitric oxide, which facilitates blood flow to the vagina. Estradiol is the type of estrogen that makes a woman feel like a woman. Estradiol has a critical impact on reproductive and sexual functioning and also acts like an antidepressant. It can effect changes in the body, including shape of bones, joints, and fat deposition, and improve arterial blood flow in coronary arteries. It is also an antioxidant that protects the brain. This hormone can be obtained with a doctor's prescription.

Estriol (E3) is one of the three main estrogens produced in the human body. It is the weakest but safest estrogen, with the fewest possible side effects to replace. Estriol is the least potent estrogen in the body and is considered to be a mild and brief-acting hormone. Estriol may protect against estrogen-associated cancers and may even help with multiple sclerosis. Studies suggest that estriol reduces symptoms of menopause, such as hot flashes and vaginal dryness, but with a better safety profile compared with more potent estrogens. It is usually applied topically in the form of a cream and is available with a doctor's prescription.

Estrogen denotes a group of hormone compounds produced primarily by developing follicles in the ovaries, the brain, and the placenta of pregnant women. Follicle-stimulating hormone (FSH) and luteinizing hormone (LH) stimulate the production of estrogen in the ovaries. Some estrogens are also produced in smaller amounts by other tissues such as the liver, adrenal glands, and the breasts. Women have more estrogen than men, which affects acetylcholine levels. This might be why women are more perceptive and intuitive. Bioidentical estrogen compounds are often helpful for treating vaginal atrophy, decreasing pain during intercourse, and improving clitoral sensitivity.

Estrone (E1) is produced by the conversion of cholesterol and found in fatty tissue. Often sold as a cream (Ogen, for example), it can be obtained with a doctor's prescription. My office does not use estrone except in very rare cases, because women are not typically deficient in this hormone. As women age, estrone usually increases, and estradiol, the predominant premenopausal estrogen, goes down. Too much estrone leads to problems including a possible risk for breast cancer. Estrone becomes the primary estrogen when the ovaries lose their function during menopause. Estrone is dependent on the production of androstenedione (an androgen) in the adrenal glands and the conversion of androstenedione to estrone, which occurs in fat tissue. This is why overweight women are at increased risk for cancers, including breast cancer.

Human growth hormone is produced by the pituitary gland. Growth hormone is critical for repair all over the body, including tissue, muscle growth, healing, brain function, immune system function, and physical and mental health, as well as bone strength. Its ability to reverse many of the major effects of aging, including muscle weakness, excess body fat deposits, energy depletion, diminished sex drive, and declining immune function, is unparalleled. Muscle growth enlivens your entire sexual experience. This can be obtained with a doctor's prescription.

Increlex is a pure form of IGF 1 (insulin growth factor). This hormone is given to women to increase muscle mass, which increases blood flow throughout the body and enhances sexual desire. It is only available by prescription.

Melatonin is produced by the pineal gland and plays a role in governing the body's circadian rhythms. It helps regulate sleep patterns, changes in body temperature, blood pressure, and heart rate. It also has antioxidant properties. It may improve sexual performance, as well as enhance serenity and relaxation after sex. Melatonin can be purchased over the counter as a supplement.

Oxytocin is produced in many different parts of the body and in the hypothalamus in the brain. Oxytocin levels rise during orgasm; supplementation can enhance orgasm contraction, leading to a more explosive and more satisfying climax; it is also the hormone that soars during child labor to allow for the birthing contractions and then allows for the bonding process between mother and child. High oxytocin levels allow for better bonding between lovers (e.g., wanting to cuddle after sex). Oxytocin also shapes memory and is the reason why many women report that they remember every detail of their child's birth, including all senses—what they saw, smelled, felt, and heard. Some women notice an increase in the size and tenderness of breast tissue while taking oxytocin. Breast and nipple massage is a natural way to increase oxytocin and therefore a very effective form of foreplay. Because of its relation to

GABA, oxytocin can also function as an antianxiety agent and can stimulate social behavior. It can be used as an antianxiety therapy and has also been used for psychiatry and autism patients very effectively for its calming and bonding effects. It is available only by prescription.

Pregnenolone is produced in the body from cholesterol. It is called the grandmother of hormones because the body uses it to create many other hormones, including DHEA and progesterone. While pregnenolone levels do not always decline with age, its by-products do, leading to illnesses and conditions like menopause. Taking pregnenolone supplements allows you to keep all your hormones at more youthful levels. Pregnenolone is the memory hormone. It also regulates GABA and serotonin levels in the brain, helping to restore the feelings of pleasure derived from sex. It can be purchased over the counter as a supplement.

Progesterone is a natural antidepressant and antianxiety agent that raises GABA. Boosting levels of this hormone in conjunction with estrogen and testosterone will help restore libido and improve mood and sleep patterns. This can be obtained with a doctor's prescription and is also available as a supplement. Progesterone is important for normal reproductive and menstrual function, and it influences the health of bone, blood vessels, heart, brain, skin, and many other tissues and organs. In addition, progesterone plays an important role in blood-sugar balance and thyroid function.

Testosterone is produced in the ovaries. It is an important component for a balanced approach to hormone replacement therapy in women. All three forms of sex hormones, including estrogen, progesterone, and testosterone, must be in proper balance with one another for optimal health. Testosterone may help women combat numerous menopausal symptoms, contributing to improvements in sexual satisfaction and orgasm as well as increased muscle mass. It also improves bone density and skin elasticity. Testosterone raises dopamine, which in turn raises sexual desire. Some women experience drastic changes in their sex lives when they start taking testosterone, including an enlarged clitoris, which facilitates greater sexual pleasure and multiple orgasms with few side effects. Yet testosterone therapy should be approached with caution and should not be used in women experiencing hair loss or excessive facial hair. Too much testosterone can convert into dihydrotestosterone, a substance that can hurt the immune system and affect appearance. When women have too much testosterone, they can gain weight, increase facial hair, and develop polycystic ovaries. A variety of natural testosterone formulations are available for women, including an injectable or a cream/gel form. Topical choices provide the easiest and most effective delivery systems, because this type of administration most closely mimics natural physiology. Testosterone is available by prescription.

Thyroid hormone (T3 and/or T4) may actually cause an underlying thyroid disease for many people with sexual dysfunction. The thyroid hormones T3 and T4 address thyroid issues. Some women positively respond to either T3 or T4, or a combination of both. These hormones can also help relieve depression, brain fog, fatigue, and other menopause-related symptoms, including difficulty losing weight. T3 is mood-elevating, which can improve your sex life, as you feel more upbeat and energetic. These can be obtained with a doctor's prescription.

Vitamin D is actually a hormone and is invaluable for improving overall health and combating menopausal symptoms, including addressing bone density loss. While your skin can manufacture some vitamin D from sunlight, most women today wear moisturizers or sunscreens, not to mention clothing, which prevent this process (you need a good portion of your skin exposed in order to really absorb vitamin D). Vitamin D comes in two forms: D_2 or D_3. I prefer D_3 because it is more effective. Either can be obtained with a doctor's prescription and are also available as over-the-counter supplements.

Nonbioidentical Hormones to Avoid:

- Birth control pills
- Cadaver growth hormones (cadaver-GH)
- Conjugated estrogens (Prempro, Premarin)
- Medroxyprogesterone (Provera)
- Methyltestosterone (Android, Testred, Virilon)

TYPICAL HORMONE DOSAGES

Dosing of hormone replacement therapy needs to be tailored to each patient's individual needs, based on his or her particular deficiencies. Most doctors who prescribe bioidentical hormones use compounding pharmacies to produce individualized dosages. The following chart shows a range of dosages and the types of delivery systems available.

HORMONAL TREATMENT	TYPICAL DOSAGE
Calcitonin • nasal spray • intramuscular injection (Miacalcin)	100–200 IU alternating nostrils daily 100 IU daily or every other day
DHEA	5–50 mg
Erythropoietin (EPO)	50–100 units/kg 3 times per week
Estradiol (E2) • transdermal gel from a compounding pharmacy • Vivelle dot patch • Climara patch	1–3 mg daily 0.025 mg–0.1 mg per day, applied twice weekly 0.025 mg–0.1 mg per day, applied weekly
Estriol (E3) Biest—combination of E3 and E2—can also be given alone	1 mg/g, apply 1–6 g per day or 5 mg/g, apply 0.5–2 g per day
Estrone (E1) Triest is a combination of all three estrogens: E1, E2, and E3	1 mg/g (E3 80%, E2 10%, E1 10%), apply 1–6 g per day
Human Growth Hormone: injection	0.05–2 mg daily
Increlex (IGF-1): injection	0.04–0.08 mg/kg twice daily
Melatonin	50 mcg–3 mg
Oxytocin • sublingual tablet • nasal spray	10–50 IU 30 minutes before intercourse 40 units/ml daily (1 spray)
Pregnenolone	10–200 mg per day
Progesterone • oral • transdermal patch	50–300 mg at bedtime Worn during menstrual cycle on days 14–25 (premenopausal) and days 1–25 (postmenopausal)
Testosterone • injection—testosterone cypionate • cream or gel	25–50 mg once per month, intramuscular 2.5–10 mg daily, applied to the skin or directly to the clitoris 30 minutes prior to intercourse
Thyroid (T3) • fast release, e.g., Cytomel • slow release from a compounding pharmacy	10–75 mcg daily 50–300 mcg daily
Thyroid (T4)	25–300 mcg daily
Vitamin D_3 (or D_2)	400 IU–10,000 IU daily or 50,000 IU once per week

New Treatment Options to Discuss with Your Doctor

Compounding pharmacies work with doctors and patients to create specialized formulations of nutrients, medications, and hormones. One such company, Bellevue Pharmacy in St. Louis, Missouri, creates combination therapies to enhance women's sexuality. These formulas contain a variety of ingredients, including prescription medications that increase blood flow to the genitals, amino acids to increase blood flow and facilitate nitric oxide synthethase (NOS), which is crucial for vaginal lubrication and genital sensation, and bioidentical hormones (often testosterone). The medications are based on generic forms of Viagra, Cialis, or Levitra, the same medications given to men for sexual dysfunction. The new therapy is then delivered vaginally. It can be used 30 minutes before intercourse to enhance sexual function.

These new therapies require a prescription, so discuss this option with your doctor to see if they are right for you.

Case Study: Alice Got Sexier When She Went Bioidentical

Alice was 59 years old when she first visited my New York City office 8 years ago. She was an active woman who traveled and exercised regularly, and she and her husband kept a jam-packed social calendar. But Alice was beginning to feel that things weren't going so well in her marriage. She was always too tired to have sex, and when she did, it was very painful. She was also having increasing difficulty falling asleep and had noticed that her skin and her hair were becoming dry.

I suspected that Alice's complaints were all related to menopause. When I mentioned this to her, she told me vehemently that she had been done with "the change" years ago, and that she was not interested in hormone replacement therapy (HRT) at this point in her life. She had read that it could have serious side effects, including cancer. But she did agree to a comprehensive workup, so that we could see definitively what was causing her condition.

Our workup confirmed that Alice was in good physical health, and her hormonal profile was within the norm for her age group. I told Alice that other doctors might be pleased with these results, but I was less than satisfied: I don't believe that we should all be resigned to sexual deterioration just because we are older. Even though she had already experienced menopause, aging was sabotaging her sex life. By enhancing her hormonal levels we could reverse her age and enhance her SexQ. I also predicted that she would see improvements in her mental acuity, and enjoy better sleep that would increase her overall energy levels.

Alice was still hesitant, but I explained how the HRT regimen I was recommending was different from the synthetic therapies she had misgivings about. The micronized hormones that I use do not contain the components used in synthetic versions that cause adverse reactions. I further explained that conventional hormone replacement therapy is frequently not balanced, such as when estrogen is given without compensating for reduced testosterone. I prescribed a micronized progesterone-estradiol-testosterone formulation, and I explained how this would boost her hormones as well as her brain chemicals.

Three months later, the change in Alice was unmistakable. She was animated as she spoke about how much younger she looked. Her skin and her hair were noticeably softer and smoother. She didn't hesitate for a moment to tell me about her renewed sex life. She was once again experiencing pleasure during sex. And she was sleeping more consistently, and finally had the energy to keep up with the many events in her day.

When I saw her again later that year, Alice remarked that along with her better overall health, she was able to concentrate better for longer periods of time. Eight years later, she is still following the same regimen, and feels much younger and sexier than what she expected to feel at 67.

Early Detection Ensures That Great Sex Lasts

By the age of 25, women typically have an estrogen-to-testosterone ratio of 20:1. A typical menopausal woman at age 48 to 52 generally comes in at 2:1, or occasionally even a 1:1 ratio. Going from a 20:1 ratio down to a 1:1 ratio would make anyone feel differently about sex. Ask your doctor to check your blood levels:

BLOOD LEVELS	TARGET RANGES
DHEA	75–125% of normal range
Estradiol	50% of normal range
Free and Total Testosterone	500
LH and FSH	Under 40 for menopausal women Under 3 for premenopausal women
Pregnenolone	75–125% of normal range
Progesterone	50% of normal range
Sex hormone binding globulin	50% of normal range
TSH	Under 2

TREATING THE SEXUAL SYMPTOMS OF MENOPAUSE

Sexually speaking, as Dr. Ruth Westheimer says, menopause is a downer. When low levels or imbalances of sex hormones occur, the ability to engage in healthy, comfortable sex is challenged. We've already discussed great techniques for improving sexual desire (Chapter 4), arousal (Chapter 5), orgasm (Chapter 6), and resolution (Chapter 7). In most instances, naturally replacing estrogen, testosterone, progesterone, and other important hormones will help these areas dramatically. You and your partner will quickly notice that your attitude toward and response to sex return to the way they were when you were younger.

The following are physical symptoms of menopause that can directly affect your sex life.

Vaginal Dryness and/or Atrophy

If you are easily aroused but cannot lubricate effectively, you may be experiencing vaginal dryness. Most perimenopausal and menopausal women are too dry. In fact, as many as 4 in 10 women who have reached menopause experience vaginal dryness. Symptoms include itching, burning, and stinging around the vaginal opening and in the lower third of the vagina, as well as the inability to lubricate during sexual intercourse. Vaginal dryness may be accompanied by pain or light bleeding during sex, urinary frequency or urgency, or an increase in frequency of urinary tract infections (UTI). Some women get UTIs from the bacteria transmitted during sex because their vaginas are too dry. The friction of sex causes an abrasion if the vagina is too dry, which can cause an infection. If you're not vaginally lubricated, you're going to go to the bathroom more often and possibly get sick.

Vaginal atrophy (atrophic vaginitis) is the thinning and inflammation of the vaginal walls, which may accompany vaginal dryness, and also involves the shortening or tightening of the vaginal canal. Both affect your ability to become sexually aroused and are caused by declining levels of estrogen as well as an acetylcholine deficiency.

The body's natural vaginal lubrication consists of clear fluid that seeps through the walls of the blood vessels encircling the vagina. When you're sexually aroused, more blood flows to your pelvic organs, creating more lubricating fluid. In order to continue to have comfortable sex, you will need to replace this lost lubrication. Using a vaginal moisturizer or water-based lubricant such as KY Jelly or Astroglide, sold at most drug stores, might help. Even better, estriol vaginal gel or Vagifem (a naturally compounded estradiol) will help create wonderful natural lubrication, so a synthetic lubricant like KY isn't even necessary. Vagifem, a vaginal estrogen tablet, can help improve the symptoms of vaginal dryness and discomfort. Vagifem is inserted into the vagina, delivering estrogen that helps the body naturally restore vaginal moisture. Avoid any product that is scented or oil-based; neither are good for the vagina and can cause further, more complicated problems.

It is also important to continue to be sexually active: The more sex you have, the more likely your own lubrication will return or continue. Sex is necessary for total vaginal health, including muscle tone and bladder tightening. You should also drink plenty of fluids each day, including water and tea.

There are a few things that you should not do if you have vaginal dryness. The first is smoking. Cigarettes and nicotine destroy estrogen in the body, so smoking only makes the problem worse. You can also make a few small changes to your personal hygiene routine. Most douches have a drying effect, which contributes to vaginal dryness, so I advise against them. Avoid using scented bath products, such as body washes and shower gels, near the vagina, and avoid bubble baths completely. These products can irritate the vagina and remove your natural lubrication if used frequently.

Lastly, when you do have sex, slow down and savor the moment. You may need more time and more physical stimulation in order to become sexually aroused, especially as you get older. Focus on foreplay, as outlined in Chapter 5, if you are finding that vaginal dryness is contributing to a lack of arousal. You might find that you and your partner are simply rushing sex and that you are not experiencing a total loss of sexual response.

Painful Intercourse (Dyspareunia)

Dyspareunia is defined as persistent or recurrent genital pain that occurs just before, during, or after intercourse and causes personal distress. Researchers at the Mayo Clinic estimate that up to 60 percent of women experience episodes of genital pain. You may have dyspareunia if you are experiencing any of the following symptoms:

- Aching pain during or after intercourse
- Burning pain during or after intercourse
- Deep pain during thrusting, described as "something being bumped"
- Pain when using tampons
- Pain with certain partners or just under certain circumstances
- Pain with penile, manual, or sex-toy penetration

Painful intercourse may be a direct result of vaginal dryness or atrophy caused by inadequate lubrication resulting from low estrogen levels. Often, this can be treated with bioidentical estrogen in either cream or tablet form like Vagifem, or estriol vaginal gel, which is available from a compounding pharmacy. In some cases, a pain medication may be necessary. Pain during sex may also be caused by medications, recent pelvic surgery, or a congenital abnormality. An infection in the genital area or urinary tract can also cause painful intercourse. Birth control products including foams, jellies, or latex from condoms, a cervical cap, or a diaphragm can all be irritating to the vagina.

Using personal lubricants and extending foreplay can help stimulate your natural lubrication, which can reduce pain. If your contraception is causing irritation or dryness, try a different preparation or talk to your doctor about switching to another type of birth control.

Lastly, broaden your sexual scope. If you experience sharp pain during thrusting, your partner's penis may be striking your cervix or stressing the pelvic floor muscles, causing aching or cramping. Try being the one on top during sex: You may be able to regulate penetration to a depth that feels better. You might also find other options beyond traditional intercourse to be more comfortable, at least until you have resolved your vaginal dryness.

Vaginismus

Involuntary spasms of the vaginal wall muscles are referred to as vaginismus, and they can make sexual penetration very painful or even impossible. Vaginismus can affect women in all stages of life, even women who have had many years of pain-free intercourse. Some women will also experience difficulty with gynecological exams or tampon insertion. Vaginismus typically follows or is triggered by temporary pelvic pain or other related problems, and can be triggered by medical conditions, traumatic events, relationship issues, surgery, or menopause. Vaginismus involves an involuntary pubococcygeus (PC) muscle contraction, which then creates a conditioned response, resulting in involuntary vaginal tightness during attempts at intercourse.

If you are experiencing these symptoms, it is important to discuss them with your spouse/partner. He should know that vaginismus is not triggered deliberately or intentionally. Left untreated, vaginismus often worsens, because the experience of ongoing sexual pain further increases its duration and intensity. Vaginismus can also impede a woman's ability to experience orgasm, as sudden pain, or the expectation of pain, derails arousal.

Traditional therapies for the symptoms of menopause—including lubrication, foreplay, and hormone supplementation—may help to resolve this issue. Another excellent treatment is the use of a vaginal dilator, which can help eliminate the PC muscle reflex associated with vaginismus.

Why Am I Eating So Much?

Increased body fat, loss of muscle tone, and gaining weight around your middle all commonly occur during menopause. The decline of estrogen and progesterone levels causes a cascade of rising blood sugars and lowered mental activity. Women feel both hungry and tired: They eat more junk food to stay alert and exercise less. The good news is that natural hormones can transform not only the way you feel, but the way you look. A diet like the one I feature in my book the *Younger (Thinner) You Diet* will also help you reach or maintain a goal of 18 to 22 percent body fat.

The dilator allows a woman to create new muscle memory as she consciously and consistently squeezes and relaxes her PC muscles with dilator insertions; eventually she learns how to override the involuntary muscle contractions that cause tightness or close the entrance to the vagina. Ultimately, the dilator helps a woman retrain her body to respond correctly to penetration so she can transition to pain-free intercourse.

CHOOSE FOODS THAT HELP YOU KEEP UP WITH YOUR MAN

Medications and supplements aren't the only ways to ramp up your sexual function. Diet is essential too. Increase your soy and fish consumption to combat all the symptoms of menopause, particularly the sexual ones. As a bonus, they will improve sexual desire and performance because they contain the building blocks of both dopamine and acetylcholine.

Fish and soy are integral parts of the Asian diet, and interestingly, Asian women experience far fewer menopausal symptoms than Western women. In one study that compared American postmenopausal women to postmenopausal Japanese women, more than 30 percent of American women complained of hot flashes, lack of energy, and depression compared with less than 10 percent of Japanese women. I believe that this is due in large part to their diets.

Fish and fish oils are loaded with essential fatty acids, which can help relieve the symptom of vaginal dryness and help retain estrogen in the body. Those highest in fatty acids are salmon, tuna, and mackerel. Non-animal sources include sesame and sunflower seeds.

Soy products contain phytoestrogens, which have both estrogen and progesterone-like properties, which is why these foods are important to include during perimenopause as well as menopause. Phytoestrogens are also found in:

- Alfalfa
- Apples
- Carrots
- Cherries
- Chickpeas
- Corn
- Flaxseeds
- Green beans
- Lemon
- Nuts
- Peas
- Potatoes
- Seeds
- Whole grains
- Yams

Soy also contains natural progesterone, as does the wild Mexican yam. Soy products also contain lignins, substances that act like estrogens and can bind to estrogen receptors. In this way, lignins can regulate your body's estrogen production. Beans, flaxseeds, and many whole grains (wheat, rice, oats, rye, millet, amaranth, quinoa, corn, barley, and buckwheat) are high in lignins.

A total of 20 to 25 grams of soy protein

per day is recommended. This translates into two to three servings of soy products daily, such as soy yogurt, soy cheese, and soy ice

SOY PRODUCT	GRAMS
Isolated soy protein (protein shake) (1 oz)	23
Soy burgers (3.2 oz)	18
Textured soy protein (tempeh) (½ cup)	11
Soy flour (1 oz)	10–13
Tofu (4 oz)	8–13
Soy milk (8 oz)	4–10

cream. Whenever possible, choose organic, as most American soy is from genetically modified organism (GMO) seeds. Soy products imported from Asia have higher potencies and yield better results.

SUPPLEMENTING YOUR SEX LIFE

While not as effective as hormone therapy for treating menopause-related symptoms or increasing sexual function, nutritional supplements are still helpful. Evening primrose oil, black currant oil, and borage oil all contain gamma-linoleic acid. Gamma-linoleic acid helps induce hormonal activity and reduces platelet aggregation, which can contribute to blocked arteries. In addition, evening primrose oil helps relieve hot flashes and may reduce heavy menstrual bleeding.

My supplement formulation called Menopause Support contains recommended potencies of the following key ingredients

that have been shown to support normal hormonal levels during menopause. This synergistic blend includes standardized herbal extracts and other nutrients that form a well-balanced and effective product for women. It contains the vitamins, minerals, and herbs that can help with menopausal symptoms associated with sex. The dosages here are suggestions if you choose to take supplements by themselves, instead of my formulation. You can choose from this list depending on your current symptoms.

Black cohosh (80–160 milligrams) may alleviate hot flashes, depression, and vaginal atrophy commonly experienced by women during menopause.

Boron (1–5 milligrams) may increase the body's levels of estradiol and testosterone, which may lead to increased sexual desire.

Calcium (500–1,000 milligrams) may help most postmenopausal women who absorb dietary calcium less efficiently and need to supplement.

Dong quai (500–2,000 milligrams) is used in traditional Chinese medicine, dong quai is often referred to as the female ginseng. It may alleviate many of the symptoms of menopause, including hot flashes and excessive perspiration.

Hops (500–2,000 milligrams) may relieve hot flashes and other menopausal discomforts.

Kava kava (200–600 milligrams) may alleviate anxiety and depression associated with menopause.

Korean (asian) ginseng (500–2,000 milligrams) may alleviate the fatigue, insomnia, and depression many menopausal women experience.

Magnesium (200–400 milligrams) keeps arteries and blood vessels relaxed, allowing for more efficient blood flow to all areas of the body, including the genitals.

Puncture vine (*Tribulus terrestris*) (250–1,000 milligrams) may alleviate many of the symptoms associated with menopause, including anxiety, apathy, depression, excessive perspiration, hot flashes, insomnia, irritability, and diminished libido.

Red clover (500–2,000 milligrams) may relieve hot flashes.

Valerian root extract (200–400 milligrams) treats insomnia, anxiety, nervous tension, and stress.

Vitex (chasteberry) (200–400 milligrams) may help to relieve hot flashes.

If You Want to Have Great Sex, These Habits Have to Go

Soda: Diet or regular, soda leeches calcium from bones, and you need all the calcium you can get

Salt: Leaves you bloated and puts you at risk for high blood pressure

Vitamins for Beating Menopause

- **DIM (diindolylmethane)** (150 milligrams twice daily) is an essential supplement for women on hormone replacement therapy. It helps estrogen metabolize safely and protects the breast.
- **Ioderal (iodine/potassium iodide)** (12.5 milligrams daily) is one of the best ways to protect and/or treat fibrocystic breasts.
- **Vitamin C** (500–5,000 milligrams), a powerful antioxidant, is great for maintaining skin tone and suppleness.
- **Vitamin E** (400–1,600 IU) is great for protecting the breasts, but it is also a blood thinner. Depending on your current health, you might not need as much.

Too Much Estrogen Makes Breasts Too Sensitive

Just as taking too much testosterone can be dangerous, oversupplementing with estrogen does not always yield a positive outcome. That's why it is so important that your bioidentical estrogen therapy be monitored by an expert physician. One side effect of too much estrogen, even when it is produced naturally by your own body, is increased sensitivity in the breasts. Swelling and tenderness result from an imbalance of estrogen and progesterone. Breast tenderness might also be a sign of breast cancer (although one can have breast cancer and not feel anything at all), or benign mastic or cystic breast tissue.

If you are experiencing pain or increased sensitivity in the breasts, see your doctor immediately. After proper screening, which can include bloodwork and mammogram/ultrasound, or MRI of the breast, the fix might be as simple as supplementing with vitamin E, iodine, or DIM. DIM is naturally found in cruciferous vegetables like cabbage, broccoli, Brussels sprouts, and cauliflower and can help guard against hormone reactive cancers, such as breast cancer. DIM stimulates more efficient estrogen metabolism, so that excess estrogen will not be stored in the body.

TREATING MENOPAUSE RESTORES TOTAL HEALTH

The menopause fix can be the first step to reversing aging in every part of your body. For example, increasing your estrogen the bioidentical way not only beats menopause and improves sexual functioning, but holds the other "pauses" at bay. Progesterone restores libido and orgasm by allowing for better relaxation; it also improves mood. Testosterone increases sex drive and also increases metabolism, controlling obesity. The chart on page 128 shows how the "big three" hormones affect the rest of the body.

It's Never Too Early—Or Too Late—To Reverse Menopause

The most important lesson any woman can take away from this book is that it is never too early or too late to start taking care of yourself. Whether you are in perimenopause or just experiencing menopausal symptoms for the first time, or menopause is years past, you can regain your health, your vitality, and your sex life. My patient Joyce is a great example of how you can take your health into your own hands at any age.

When Joyce first came to see me 5 years ago, she was tired of everything in her life. She had gone through menopause 10 years earlier at the age of 53, and in the first year after she stopped menstruating, she gained 80 pounds. Most women would find that reasonably upsetting, but Joyce was incensed: She had been a dancer all her life and couldn't believe the body she now inhabited. Eventually she had become resigned to her new weight, but she couldn't accept losing her memory.

I ran my routine of tests and uncovered Joyce's complete medical history. Together, we decided to aggressively treat her aging. Joyce had chosen not to take the hormones that her gynecologist had offered because she read that they caused cancer, but she instantly understood the difference between them and the bioidenticals I recommended. I prescribed testosterone cream to boost her sexuality; Biest cream and progesterone to balance her hormone levels to a younger state and return her memory; HGH to improve her bones and her muscle mass; thyroid hormone to give her energy; Klonopin to help her sleep at night; and Wellbutrin to keep her from becoming anxious during the day. She also injected Forteo for the first 2 years to prevent osteoporosis and is maintaining the results with calcitonin.

In 1 year she lost all the weight she had gained in the past 10 years. Five years later, I'm still making small adjustments to her individualized program with preventive measures, and when something comes up, we address it quickly and decisively.

Joyce is now back to her old life of travel and lots of dancing. She told me, "I am constantly told that I look like I could be in my late forties. Nobody believes that I'm 69 years old. I have a fabulous life. After the past 5 years of treatment, I feel like a completely new woman: head to toe! I thought menopause was the end, but for me, it's been the beginning of a whole new life."

You can craft a preventive medicine program that's specific to your needs. By following my protocol outlined in the rest of the book, you'll learn more about the relationship between sex and the other pauses, as well as the diet and exercise program you'll need to follow to achieve your very best SexQ.

Benefits of the Big Three Hormones

	ESTROGEN	PROGESTERONE	TESTOSTERONE
Dopamine function	Decreases storage of body fat	Helps increase appetite, acts as a natural diuretic, and helps stabilize blood sugar levels	Helps weight loss
Acetylcholine function	Improves memory and cognitive abilities	Calms the mind	Improves visual spatial memory and working memory
GABA function	Reduces anxiety attacks, improves mood	Reverses seizures and anxiety	Reduces anxious behaviors
Serotonin function	Improves sleep patterns	Improves sleep patterns	Improves sleep patterns
Cardiopause	Improves heart function	Lowers blood pressure, prevents arrhythmias	Helps heart pump more efficiently
Dermatopause	Increases radiance and hydration in skin, hair, and nails	Keeps skin supple	Keeps skin moist
Immunopause	Decreases risk of breast cancer	Prevents breast and endometrial cancers and possibly other cancers	Most cancers increase as testosterone decreases with age.
Osteopause	Improves bone density	Stimulates bone density	Improves hip bone density
Thyropause	Improves thyroid function	Improves thyroid function	Improves thyroid function
Vasculopause	Improves blood flow, decreases blood clotting	Improves circulation	Increases blood flow

PART III

Younger (Sexier) You for Men

CHAPTER 9

Beat Male Menopause and Enhance Your SexQ

THE TYPICAL HIGH-DOPAMINE male is sexually autistic—his one-track mind is governed by a combination of testosterone and his SexQ. When your SexQ is high dopamine, you need to have lots of sex, because you have lots of physical energy. When you are high acetylcholine, you have a romantic streak that could give Casanova a run for his money. If you are high GABA, then you're lucky because you can manipulate your sex drive to match your spouse's. But if you are high serotonin, your spouse may not understand your need to wander.

Unfortunately, these highs don't last forever. As we age, brain chemistry dwindles. What was once a high SexQ will eventually turn into a lower one. I can't tell you how many men have come to see me when they were having sex as few as four times a year. While this change doesn't happen overnight, a declining sexuality is slow and steady. The good news is that once these men do seek medical attention, in just a few months I get them to a place where they are having sex four times a week and loving it. Whether they are 30 or 80, I've seen men who haven't had sex for 9 years who can now have sex whenever they want to, and believe me, they want to.

The fix usually involves creating more testosterone. An estimated 5 million American men have a medical condition called hypogonadism, or low testosterone, while others have simply lost testosterone as they aged. Your frequency of orgasm is telling. When you were in your teens, you might have had wet dreams, which were nothing more than orgasms occurring during sleep. During your twenties, your sex life becomes more controlled: Testosterone levels were still high but already falling, around 1,000 ng/dl (nanograms per deciliter). By age 30, they have dropped to around 900, and decrease every year after that. By the time they decline as low as 300, men are sexually wasted.

Your Sexuality Ages Faster Than the Rest of You

TESTOSTERONE LEVELS (NG/DL)	AGE
1,000	20
900	30
800	40
700	50
600	60
500	70
400	80
300	90
200	100

SIGNS AND SYMPTOMS THAT YOUR TESTOSTERONE LEVELS ARE FALLING

Aside from sexual function, low testosterone levels affect your overall health. Here are a few other warning signs of dwindling testosterone.

- Anxiety
- Decline in general well-being
- Decreased beard growth
- Decreased hair and nail growth
- Depressed mood
- Excessive sweating
- Fatigue
- Irritability
- Joint pain and muscle achiness
- Loss of skin elasticity
- Loss of vitality
- Nervousness
- Sleep disturbances or problems

Have You Heard of Andropause?

Testosterone loss is the hallmark of andropause, the male equivalent of menopause. Andropause affects every aspect of sex, from desire to performance. It also can affect your mood, memory and thinking, and most of all, your health. The loss of testosterone also results in low satisfaction, from motivation and drive, from engaging in activities you once found enjoyable, including sex.

Andropause typically begins at age 40, but it can occur earlier in life if you are under enormous stress, have episodes of depression, or use recreational drugs. However, andropause is much more flexible than menopause: Testosterone levels can naturally rebound with the right lifestyle changes and supplementation. Even if you

Lack of Sex Puts You in a Bad Mood

Without testosterone, men run the risk of becoming cantankerous old coots who throw temperamental fits. The loss of hormones leads to bickering and alienation because you've essentially been neutered—no longer "man" enough to feel good about yourself. These feelings may lead you to take out that anger and frustration on your family.

are losing testosterone due to natural aging, you can still replace this hormone, and others, for optimal health. Indeed, it's important to do so because the hormone component of becoming younger and sexier is worth 20 to 30 more years of good sex.

Some of the sexual symptoms of andropause include:

- Decline in penis length and scrotum size
- Decreased sexual desire
- Decreased sexual arousal
- Decreased intensity of orgasm
- Premature ejaculation
- Erectile dysfunction

Testosterone vs. Viagra

There has been an explosion of erectile drugs on the market for men who need a little extra help. The tremendous volume of sales demonstrates the magnitude of this problem. It's a shame that men have fallen into the pharmaceutical trap of believing the only way to fix their problem is with a prescription. They are willing to risk serious side effects rather than seek alternative methods.

Changes to your libido, or sex drive, are controlled by dopamine and testosterone. Consequently, with my patients I have found that male sexual dysfunction is more effectively treated with testosterone supplementation than Viagra. Viagra addresses specific health issues related to sexual performance; if you do not have penile blood flow or circulatory issues, you don't need Viagra (more on this in Chapter 10). And in general when men get more testosterone, they don't need Viagra either. The bottom line is that you don't have to take a drug if you can fix your dopamine levels and adjust your metabolism and libido. The use of these drugs over the long term isn't healthy because the side effects are wide-ranging.

If Men Only Had More Estrogen

One reason that women live longer than men might be that women have more estrogen. Estrogen receptors increase the expression of longevity-associated genes. Plant-based phytoestrogens, found in soy and wine, may be beneficial for men when estrogen replacement therapy is not: Estrogen supplements are too feminizing for men. On the other hand, men don't lose as much estrogen, so they aren't at risk of losing cognitive ability as many women do during menopause.

THE BEST SEX REQUIRES NATURAL BIOIDENTICAL HORMONES

All of your hormones play some role in healthy sexual function. Your brain sends its electrical signals as hormonal messengers to your aging testes, liver, thyroid, pituitary and adrenal glands, and many other organs to give them an additional jump start. As we get older, the brain needs to send more of these chemical messengers to get the same job done, the result of which is ultimately toxic to your brain. As we age, hormones such as FSH and luteinizing hormone increase in a desperate attempt to stimulate sexual organs. These two hormones can accelerate dementia and create other health problems. By enhancing the right hormone levels through supplementation, your natural levels of FSH and luteinizing hormones remain low. At the same time, you are providing your brain and body with the right balance of hormones to keep you younger and sexier.

Men have been taking testosterone replacements since the mid-1930s, but today's formulations are significantly improved. Naturally micronized testosterones and other hormones safely treat hypogonadism as well as andropause by restoring testosterone to its normal range. I have been using testosterone and growth hormone replacement therapies for my male patients for more than 10 years, enabling these men to maintain brain function as well as sexual stamina and libido.

Natural testosterone is available in many different forms, including pills, pellets, creams, patches, injectables, and gels that you simply rub into your skin, including the commonly prescribed Androgel pump. In my office we find that it's better to compound testosterone gel to a patient's individual needs rather than use a cookie-cutter formulation. A study reported in the *Journals of Gerontology* showed that men 65 to 87 who used testosterone transdermal patches for 1 year also improved their memory and concentration abilities.

However, not all hormone therapies are created equal. For example, the synthetic methyltestosterone now carries a warning of liver cancer. Other complications associated with synthetic progesterone include weight gain, heart disease, and stroke. It has also been shown that growth hormone derived from cadavers causes cancer. I only prescribe bioidentical hormones, which are plant-based, natural, and safe. These compounds have precisely the same molecular structure as those made in the human body, so they produce the same physiologic responses as the body's own hormones. Bioidentical hormones have been available for more than 20 years. They are so free from side effects that they are frequently sold over the counter as nutrient supplements (melatonin, pregnenolone, vitamin D_3, and DHEA to name a few). They offer an effective way to alleviate symptoms of andropause without introducing dangerous, synthetic toxins into your already taxed body. At the same time, these bio-identical hormones will jump-start your brain's chemical production, especially of dopamine and acetylcholine, which is exactly what you need to increase your sex drive.

There is a wide range of bioidentical hormones that you can consider replacing, depending on your current health status. Many work together. I have found that my patients who take a combination of bio-identical growth hormone and testosterone show the best results. For example, Don was 55 and both discouraged and depressed about his sexual dysfunction. I changed his antidepressant and started him on my sexual rejuvenation hormone program. He went from having sex with his wife once per month to six times per week!

The Best of the Bioidenticals

Read through the following list carefully, and discuss with your doctor which of these preparations is right for you.

Aldosterone is a hormone that regulates sodium and potassium levels as well as maintains appropriate blood volumes, and may have a protective effect on hearing. Fluids and proper levels of sodium and potassium are essential for inner ear nerve signaling to the brain—a process critical for normal hearing. Researchers discovered that people with age-related hearing loss may have only half of the aldosterone they need. It is available with a doctor's prescription.

Calcitonin is produced by the thyroid gland and affects bone growth and calcium regulation. It is generally administered as a nasal spray or through injection. It can be obtained with a doctor's prescription.

DHEA is produced in the adrenal glands, the adrenal cortex, and the brain as well as the testes in men. It is then converted to estrogen and testosterone. Reestablishing DHEA balance to original youthful levels can enhance sexual desire, receptivity, and performance and restore the pleasure derived from sex. It is also used for chronic fatigue syndrome, depression, memory loss, osteoporosis, and to protect the body from the ravages of age. Watch for products with labels indicating they contain "7 Keto DHEA." This formulation does not convert or metabolize into testosterone in the same way as DHEA. However, there are many studies that show it improves the immune system and cuts down on gut fat. It can be purchased over the counter as a supplement.

Erythropoietin (EPO) is produced by the kidneys and is the hormone that regulates red blood cell production in the bone marrow. It is used to treat anemia and has been studied for its ability to improve libido. It can also be used as a way to improve sexual functioning for men who suffer from scleroderma, a condition of extremely tight, hard skin. This bioidentical hormone can be obtained with a doctor's prescription.

Human growth hormone (HGH) is produced by the pituitary gland. Growth hormone is critical for repair all over the body, including tissue, muscle growth, healing, brain function, immune system function, and physical and mental health, as well as bone strength. Its ability to reverse many of the major effects of aging, including muscle weakness, excess body fat deposits, energy depletion, and declining immune function, is unparalleled. It can also help boost a reduced sex drive. This can be obtained with a doctor's prescription.

Melatonin is produced by the pineal gland and plays a role in governing the body's circadian rhythms. It helps regulate sleep patterns, changes in body temperature, blood pressure, and heart rate. It also has antioxidant properties. It may improve sexual performance, as well as enhance serenity and relaxation after sex. Melatonin can be purchased over the counter as a supplement.

Oxytocin is only produced in the male brain's hypothalamus. It has the ability to increase libido, as well as the desire to cuddle or be held. Oxytocin may make men feel more romantic. Because of its relation to GABA, oxytocin can also function as an antianxiety agent and can stimulate social behavior. It is available only by prescription.

Pregnenolone is produced in the body from cholesterol. It is called the grandmother of hormones because the body uses it to create many other hormones, including testosterone, cortisone, progesterone, DHEA, and others. Taking pregnenolone supplements allows you to keep all your hormones at more youthful levels. Pregnenolone regulates GABA and serotonin levels in the brain, helping to restore the feelings of pleasure derived from sex. Pregnenolone can be purchased over the counter as a supplement.

Progesterone is a natural antidepressant and tranquilizer that raises GABA. Boosting levels of this hormone in conjunction with testosterone will help restore libido and improve mood and sleep patterns. Progesterone makes men become less aggressive, can help them feel more sexual, and can shrink the prostate. It can be obtained as a supplement.

Prostaglandin E (alprostadil/ MUSE) helps relax muscle tissue in the penis, which enhances the blood flow needed for erection. There are two ways to administer this medication: Needle-injection therapy allows you to use a fine needle to inject the hormone into the base or side of your penis. This generally produces an erection in 5 to 20 minutes and lasts about an hour. A second delivery method uses a disposable applicator to insert a tiny suppository, about half the size of a grain of rice, into the tip of the penis. The suppository is absorbed by the erectile tissue, increasing blood flow and causing an erection. These hormone-delivery therapies are only available with a prescription.

Testosterone therapy has been shown to produce significant improvements in sexual satisfaction and orgasm. Testosterone increases dopamine, which raises sexual desire. It is also known to elevate brain function, increase muscle mass, and improve physical stamina.

Studies also show that restoring male testosterone balance can improve memory and concentration. Testosterone also regulates the brain's dopamine and leptin levels, which keeps men trim. Topical testosterone (along with prostaglandin) has been shown to help some men with ED. Yet testosterone therapy should be approached with caution, because there are serious side effects (see Chapter 4 for more details). A variety of natural testosterone formulations are available in injectable, pill, cream, patch, or gel form. Topical creams provide the easiest and most effective delivery systems. Testosterone is available by prescription.

Thyroid hormone (T3 and/or T4) Many men with sexual dysfunction may actually have underlying thyroid disease that has not been properly diagnosed. Many men respond better to a combination of T4 (thyroxine) and T3 (triiodothyronine). These hormones can also help relieve depression, brain fog, fatigue, and other age-related symptoms. T3 is mood-elevating, which may be why it is thought to improve your sex life as you feel more energetic. It is obtained with a doctor's prescription.

Vasopressin may increase romantic feelings and improve memory. It's important to rebalance the hormone vasopressin if you have an issue with frequent urination after sex. This bioidentical hormone is commonly used to control bed-wetting in children, and it may help adults as well. It is obtained with a doctor's prescription.

Vitamin D$_3$ is invaluable for strengthening overall health. While your skin can manufacture some vitamin D from sunlight, you may wear moisturizers or sunscreens that prevent this process. It can be obtained with a doctor's prescription and is also available as an over-the-counter supplement.

Typical Hormone Dosages

HORMONAL TREATMENT	TYPICAL DOSAGE
Aldosterone	50–200 mcg daily
Calcitonin • nasal spray • intramuscular injection	100–200 IU alternating nostrils daily 100 IU daily or every other day
DHEA	25–100 mg daily
Erythropoietin (EPO)	50–100 units/kg 3 times per week
Human Growth Hormone: injection	0.05–2 mg daily
Melatonin	0.5–3 mg per day, fast-release 1–5 mg per day, slow-release
Oxytocin • sublingual tablet • nasal spray	10–50 IU 30 minutes before intercourse 40 units/ml daily (1 spray)

(continued)

(continued)

HORMONAL TREATMENT	TYPICAL DOSAGE
Pregnenolone	10–200 mg daily
Progesterone	50–300 mg at bedtime daily
Prostaglandin E	5–40 mcg daily as needed
Testosterone	50–150 mg daily
Thyroid (T3) • fast-release, e.g., Cytomel • slow-release	10–75 mcg daily 50–300 mcg daily
Thyroid (T4)	25–300 mcg daily
Vasopressin	0.25–0.5 ml, 2–3 times daily as needed
Vitamin D_3	400–10,000 IU daily or 50,000 IU once per week

Case Study: Thomas Didn't Need Viagra After All

Thomas is one of my most remarkable medical reversal stories. He came to see me when he was just 46 years old, and I have never met a braver man. Thomas was a member of the New York City Police Department and served during 9/11, so when Tom came in asking for Viagra, I wanted to give something back to him—not just a healthy penis. Tests revealed that Tom was suffering from hypogonadism, or low testosterone. Additionally, the stress from his job was taking a toll on his health: He was experiencing depression, high blood pressure, and chronic exhaustion. Surprisingly, Tom had been willing to live with all of these symptoms, but when sexual dysfunction was added to the list, it pushed him over the edge. His erectile dysfunction compounded his depression, finally forcing Tom off the couch and into my office.

The full medical history and brain health quiz revealed that Tom's brain was imbalanced: His serotonin levels were way down. So before we rushed to the Viagra samples, I told Tom that we should try to fix his brain first.

Get Used to New Hormone Levels

I once prescribed testosterone to a married clergyman, only to have him return to my office less than a week later complaining that he was overcome by the desire to fondle his wife, along with his female congregants. He was shocked and upset and demanded, "What is wrong with me? I'm lusting after everybody!" I assured him that he wasn't going through a crisis of faith, just adjusting to his new SexQ. Sometimes, you need to adjust your prescription or learn to intellectually manage your changing brain chemistry. That's why you need to work with a doctor who prescribes these medications regularly. If your doctor is new to this treatment protocol, you might want to get a referral to someone else more experienced.

Sex Depends on Healthy Cartilage

The penis is made of cartilage. The hormones T3 (thyroid hormone) and growth hormone can increase the mass and weight of cartilage.

I immediately put Tom on the antidepressant Effexor, which solved several problems at the same time. Not only did his mood improve, but his sexual function was restored, simply by enhancing his brain chemistry. He was also able to stop feeding his bad mood with bad foods, and he lost almost 30 pounds in the first 6 months of treatment. We boosted his SexQ with DHEA and vitamin D_3. Tom now feels like the hero he always was, especially to his wife.

YOUR HEALTH CAN BE AFFECTING YOUR SEX LIFE

Diseases of the body can adversely affect your sexuality. Obesity is one of the worst age accelerators for men, with alcohol and drug abuse not far behind. More than 70 percent of men who suffer from sexual dysfunction can trace their issues to cardiovascular disease, hypertension, diabetes, depression, stress-related illnesses, or associated medications.

Take the case of Mel, a 60-year-old patient who had not had an erection since suffering a heart attack 9 years earlier. After losing more than 40 pounds and going on my hormone revitalization program consisting of growth hormone, natural testosterone, and DHEA, he regained his ability to repeatedly achieve orgasm.

SEX SAVES YOUR PROSTATE

Prostate cancer is not a sexually transmitted disease. In fact, the more ejaculations one has, the better. Frequent sex decreases the risk of prostate cancer by as much as 33 percent. Prostate cancer in most cases is genetic, and there is a high prevalence of prostate cancer in men with low testosterone levels.

The prostate is a walnut-size gland that lies between the bladder and the penis, and it is vitally important to every man's health and sexual performance. The prostate carries urine from the bladder and adds fluid to sperm just before ejaculation. Painful urination postorgasm is a sign of a prostrate problem, or what is often described as LUTS: lower urinary tract symptoms. Sex is a stress test on your prostate and urethra. If your prostate isn't healthy, you're going to find that you are urinating very often, and you may get sick.

Benign prostatic hyperplasia (BPH) can begin as early as age 30, although most men will not experience symptoms until they reach their fifties. Prostatitis is a bacterial infection of the prostate that can occur at any age and is quickly remedied by antibiotics. Prostatic hypertrophy, or enlargement of the prostate, is another common prostate problem unrelated to prostate cancer. It is estimated that 70 percent of men over age 50 have some prostatic enlargement.

Prostate cancer is second only to lung cancer as the most common form of cancer among American men. Symptoms of this slow-moving disease include painful urination, bone pain, and nodules on the prostate that may be felt during a digital rectal exam.

If prostate problems persist, surgery may be required. A common sexual side effect is orgasm without ejaculation. The key, of course, is to help prevent prostate problems from developing by catching these diseases as early as possible. See your doctor if you experience the following symptoms:

- Painful urination with lower back pain, fever, and/or pelvic pain
- An urge to urinate but inability to get a stream started
- Weak urine stream
- Frequent urination
- Sensation of full bladder after urination

Your Prostate Needs to Be Monitored

After age 50, your prostate should be monitored during your annual doctor's visit. Men should receive yearly ultrasounds on the prostate, just as women have annual mammograms. Other tests for prostate health include:

- Bloodwork to determine testosterone level and PSA (prostate-specific antigen)
- Digital rectal exams

- PAP: prostate acid phosphatase testing
- PET scans

Natural Treatments for Prostate Problems

There are several natural treatments available for prostate cancer and benign prostatic hypertrophy (BPH) that, if used early, can reverse the problems.

- **Bee/flower pollen (cernilton)** has been reported to improve symptoms of BPH.
- **Beta-sitosterol** is a compound found to assist in urinary flow.
- **Citrus pectin** has been shown to shrink the prostate gland.
- **Garlic** in heavy consumption was shown in a University of Hong Kong study to decrease the incidence of prostate cancer.
- **Glycine, alanine, and glutamic acid compound** is one supplement that contains all three amino acids. It has been proven to reduce swelling in the prostate.
- **Lycopene** is found in watermelon and tomatoes. This nutrient can reduce the risk of prostate cancer by more than 40 percent. You need to have 10 servings a week of tomatoes in order to have a strong anticancer effect.
- **Pumpkin seeds** contain essential fatty acids that can protect the prostate.
- **Pygeum** is an herb native to Africa that has been clinically proven to alleviate BPH. Taken with saw palmetto, the

Exercise Helps the Prostate

Exercising has been found to lower the risk of prostate problems. However, bike riding may cause enlargement of the prostate, so if you experience any of the symptoms listed, try to avoid this form of exercise if possible.

combination of these two herbs may reduce prostate issues and has been shown to reverse impotence.

- **Saw palmetto** contains fatty acids, esters, and sterols that keep the prostate healthy and reduce inflammation.
- **Vitamin C** in high doses may decrease prostate toxicity and reduce the possibility of cancer.
- **Vitamin E** in its gamma form may be very effective in helping men avoid prostate cancer. Make sure to purchase vitamin E as a mixed formula that contains the

gamma version, or buy gamma tocopherol separately.

- **Zinc** has been shown to reduce the size of the prostate.

Prevent the Dreaded Droop

There's plenty you can do to create more testosterone naturally. One of the best places to start is in the kitchen. In order to reverse andropause, you need to create as much testosterone and dopamine from the foods you choose. Vitamin C–rich foods like beet

Andropause Plus Addiction Kills Your Chances for Great Sex

Addiction and andropause often go together, creating what I call reward deficiency syndrome. Vices are often attempts at self-medicating. Whether it's eating too many doughnuts, drinking too much coffee, or taking prescription or recreational drugs, the addiction is the same. The brain creates a craving in an escalating attempt to find reward as dopamine levels decline.

Alcohol is a particularly poor choice. Night after night of one too many can dull the nerves that transmit sensation between your penis and brain. Research at Southern Illinois University found that having more than eight drinks three times a week causes a drop in every measure of arousal. For example, I once treated a prominent 54-year-old attorney whose dopamine was so out of whack that he was abusing cocaine, binge drinking every night, and hiring high-priced prostitutes. Yet once he bedded each "escort," he found that he could not perform. Even Viagra and Cialis didn't do the job.

His bloodwork showed that his problem was a combination of diabetes and deficiencies in both testosterone and growth hormone. He also had chronic anxiety and panic attacks due to low levels of GABA. I put him on a therapy program of niacin, fish oil, natural testosterone, DHEA, and growth hormone. Within 2 months he was having three erections a week and staying home with his wife. Better still, he was off alcohol and cocaine. By balancing his brain by improving his mood and reducing his anxiety, I was able to cure his addiction and restore his SexQ.

Younger, Sexier Women Prefer Men with Hair

Foods that are high in copper and zinc aid hair growth. Choose barley, beets, garlic, nuts, pecans, radishes, raisins, seafood, and soy. Fish provides essential fatty acids that keep hair healthy.

greens, black currants, mangoes, sweet peppers, and pineapples can improve stamina and circulation. Zinc supplementation may be necessary: A deficiency may be an underlying case of lowered sexual desire. Follow the dopamine diet outlined in Chapter 4 by focusing on tyrosine- and phenylalanine-rich foods seasoned with oregano and rosemary for an added dopamine punch.

Then, get yourself to the gym, and focus on strength training that increases your muscles. According to Oslo University studies, this can produce a 20 percent testosterone surge in just 3 months. Another important exercise can be done anywhere: the infamous Kegel. As women know, Kegels boost circulation and strengthen your groin muscles.

Next, get into bed, but don't go to sleep. Researchers who followed 1,000 men ages 55 to 75 for 5 years found that those who had sex less than once a week at the start of the study were twice as likely to develop erectile dysfunction (ED) as those who had it at least once a week. As for the even livelier older men who had sex three or more times a week, they lowered their risk fourfold.

Last, get a good night's sleep. Besides boosting serotonin, sleep allows your brain and your penis to reset. Believe it or not, while you sleep, you have between three and five hour-long erections. These erections are a good sign that your circulatory system is working (thus putting the Viagra idea out of your head).

Don't Overthink Sexual Performance

I've found that almost a third of my ED patients are suffering from self-fulfilling overexpectation. Any preoccupation with penile performance blocks out the erotic thoughts you need to get going. If you have no problem during masturbation, it's more than likely that there's nothing physically wrong. Relax and you'll rise to the occasion soon enough.

During sex, train your mind to think of something other than ejaculation. Focusing on a phrase like "I don't want to ejaculate" is still thinking about ejaculation. I don't recommend reciting sports statistics either: Both of these techniques will only divert your attention from your partner. It is essential that you be fully present in order to relax enough to maintain your erection. Instead of thinking about ejaculation or worrying about ejaculating too quickly, I suggest you think about pleasing your partner. If you concentrate on what she likes, you'll find that you get what you want as well.

When Size Matters

The loss of growth hormone, testosterone, and many of the other hormones we've discussed in this chapter will inevitably lead to a loss of penis size. In fact, men lose 20 percent of their erection size with age. But many men are needlessly worried about what I call midget penis syndrome. Most men underestimate the size of their penis, leaving 86 percent of men feeling that they don't measure up. Who needs this kind of performance anxiety? In a study at the University of Pittsburgh, 26 percent of men gauged their own penis size as below average. The problem, however, is that they are not measuring properly. First, stop looking at your penis from above. From that vantage point, even your stomach looks small.

Grab a tape measure and a ruler. To check your flaccid length, measure it quickly: A cold or warm room can cause shrinkage or growth. Position the tip of the ruler where the shaft meets the abdomen, then place the ruler along the shaft and read the length. An average length is 3.43 inches.

Measure your erection as soon as you are hard. Start at the side farthest from your testicles and measure to the tip of your shaft, holding the ruler against your penis base. An average length is 5.03 inches. Now wrap the tape measure around your penis at its base. An average girth is 5.14 inches.

If you measure up but still feel small,

testosterone and growth hormone supplementation may enlarge you to some degree. Or you can create an illusion of having a bigger penis by trimming your pubic hair. Losing weight doesn't hurt, either; heavy-set and obese men gain weight through their pelvic regions, making their penises look smaller than they actually are. You can also rub on a lotion that contains arginine, which will temporarily increase the size of blood vessels on the penis, causing the tissue to enlarge more fully during erection.

The Night Stalker

Your erectile dysfunction may be nothing more than performance anxiety. One way to check is to see if you are having erections during sleep, which most men experience without even realizing. In my office I test men who experience erectile dysfunction with a standard nocturnal penile tumescence (NPT) test that they

Don't Even Think about It

You've seen the ads in magazines or on Web sites that tout pills or techniques to make you larger, but none of these has been clinically proven to work.
- Clamping
- Jelqing (a.k.a. milking; pulling the penis away from one's body)
- Penis enlargement pills
- Penis patches
- Penis pump

Penile Erection Preservative

Some men with ED need a little "PEP," or "penile erection preservative." They are treated with the same antidepressants that can cause others to have a secondary sexual dysfunction. One common source of low libido and changes in sexual performance is the use of antidepressants known as selective serotonin reuptake inhibitors. Antidepressants such as Prozac and Zoloft are among the most widely prescribed treatments for depression, and they often create a drop in sex drive or anorgasmia, which happens when desire is there but you can't orgasm. But for men with ED, lowering your speed of orgasm might be exactly what you need to succeed.

perform at home over a 3-day period. The test uses a small, portable computer connected to two bands placed around the shaft of the penis; the computer monitors changes in the penis and can detect and record the presence of an erection occurring during sleep.

You can perform a similarly effective NPT test the old-fashioned way, with a roll of stamps. Simply tape a strip of stamps snugly around the shaft of your flaccid penis before you go to bed. If the strip breaks at night, it means that you had an erection and you are physically capable of having an erection during sex. If you can experience an erection while sleeping but cannot obtain one while awake, a psychological cause or a medication side effect is to blame. But if you can't obtain an erection either awake or in the sleeping state, there is generally a physiological cause.

IMPROVE SEXUAL PERFORMANCE

There are a host of exercises you can work on that can improve your sexual timing and raise your serotonin. These exercises can be done before, during, or after sex.

Just say "Om": The secret to preventing premature ejaculation and having marathon sex may lie in the ancient art of yoga. Studies from the International Society for Sexual Medicine found that men who performed yoga poses several times a day took longer to ejaculate than men who did not. I would deduce that yoga is equally effective for improving women's timing, as yoga helps us get in touch with the workings of the body. The more physically flexible and relaxed you can become, the easier it will be to get into a sexual position that works wonders for you.

Squeeze play: Apply firm pressure with the thumb and forefinger on the urethra—the tube that runs along the underside of the penis. This technique can momentarily decrease sexual tension, preventing ejaculation.

Don't go "all the way": During sex focus on small, shallow movements that penetrate the first 2 to 3 inches of the vaginal canal. You'll last longer if you're not thrusting vigorously. And, this movement might be just the thing to hit your partner's G-spot, causing greater arousal.

Keep the Kegels coming: Kegels help tighten the pubococcygeal (PC) muscles of the pelvic floor. To find your PC muscle, try cutting off the flow of urine when peeing. Once you have better control of those muscles, you can engage them during sex, squeezing your pelvic floor muscles around the scrotum, penis, and anus when you feel ejaculation approaching.

Taoist advanced Kegels: Squeeze your PC muscles, roll your eyes upward, touch your tongue to the roof of your mouth, and visualize your sexual energy flowing up through your body. And practice controlled breathing, too. Sounds complicated, but I've found that this is one of the most effective ways of delaying ejaculation.

Pressure your perineum: The perineum is located midway between the scrotum and the anus, and putting a small amount of pressure here will help delay ejaculation. That's because this spot reaches through to the prostate gland, which contracts and expands during orgasm and expels ejaculate. The prostate feels like a bumpy walnut shape beneath your fingers. You or your partner can stimulate it by lightly massaging the perineum in a circular motion, first clockwise and then counterclockwise. Ask your partner to apply this pressure for you, or do it yourself for more control.

Tug your testes: When a man nears orgasm, his scrotum rises up closer to the body. You or your partner can delay ejaculation by gently pulling the testes down and away from the body.

Suicide squeeze: Squeezing the penis just below the head, or glans, can help stop ejac-ulation. It requires that you withdraw completely from your partner, which will also help intercourse last longer.

Mind games: Focus on moving your sexual energy through your body. Stopping movement, relaxing a little, and taking deep, slow breaths go a long way.

Stop Yelling: Hearing Loss Affects Your Sex Life

Hearing loss is a common problem for men, and it may affect their sex lives. No one wants to have sex with someone they have to scream at in order to be heard. And you may be missing lots of whispers and verbal foreplay if you can't hear what your partner is saying. A study from San Diego, California, found that men are 2.5 times more likely to develop noise-induced hearing loss (NIHL) than women. Occupational and recreational noise exposure, including power tools, lawn mowers, leaf blowers, motorcycles, and

A Younger, Sexier Thrusting Technique

Combine deep and shallow thrusts for more staying power. Deep thrusts allow the penis to penetrate completely. Shallow thrusts mean that the penis only enters 1½ to 2 inches inside the vagina. For every nine quick shallow thrusts, allow one slow deep one. The shallow thrusts stimulate the most sensitive vaginal tissues and create a vacuum effect that makes your partner eager for the deep thrust to come. And when most of your thrusts are affecting only the first few inches of your penis, you'll be able to last much longer.

hunting, as well as service in the armed forces, may be some factors that put men at greater risk.

There is increasing evidence that NIHL can lead to temporary or permanent hearing loss. Hearing receptor cells in the inner ear, called hair cells, are normally stimulated by sound waves that cause the eardrum and bones of hearing to vibrate. These vibrations are sent to the brain, where they are translated. However, excessively loud sounds can cause extreme deformation and permanent damage to these hair cells. Worse, these hair cells are nonrenewable; damage can be permanent.

One of the easiest ways to prevent hearing loss goes against the cultural norm of today: Banish the ubiquitous personal music players. The highest acceptable industrial noise exposure level is 115 decibels for 15 minutes a day: These devices can produce sounds of up to 130 decibels, enough to cause permanent damage. Do yourself, and your screaming spouse, a favor by turning down your MP3 to 60 percent of total volume. Or invest in a pair of speakers so you both can get into the groove.

BREAK ANDROPAUSE FOR A YOUNGER (SEXIER) YOU

It's relatively easy to get your groove back on. A multimodal approach that includes medications, hormones, nutrient supplements, and specific dietary suggestions will help. The first step is to make certain you are treating the disease, instead of the symptoms.

Your physician might recommend some of the following bloodwork, as well as a prostate ultrasound and penile Doppler. Prostate, bladder, and kidney health can all be easily investigated using ultrasound technology, which tends to be more accurate than a manual exam (not to mention more comfortable).

The rest of the book will help you craft a preventive medicine program that's specific to your needs. You'll learn more about the relationship between sex and the other "pauses," as well as the right diet and exercise program you'll need to follow to achieve your very best SexQ. First, learn more about circulatory issues pertaining to your sex life, and discover if prescription medications such as Viagra are really indicated.

Know Your Ratios

For young men, testosterone-to-estrogen levels should be around 20:1. As we age, these levels shift. Unlike women, however, when a man's testosterone drops, he does not experience as drastic a fluctuation in hormonal levels. Men's ratios generally bottom out at about 6:1, one reason why the symptoms of andropause are less severe than the symptoms of menopause.

Blood Tests Every Man Should Have

LH and FSH	Measures the brain's electrical/chemical messenger to the testicles. 50% of men in andropause have high LH or FSH, and 50% have low or normal levels.
Prostate-specific antigen (PSA)	Screening for prostate cancer
Sex hormone–binding globulin	A key modulator between male and female sexual hormones. This test identifies male menopause.
Testosterone free and total	There are two kinds of testosterone in the body; total is the reserve, and free is what the body is using.

CHAPTER 10

The Total Sex Checkup for Men

ERECTILE DYSFUNCTION (ED) IS complex and far reaching. There are seven major categories of sexual dysfunction, ranging from desire disorders, arousal disorders, orgasm disorders, sexual pain disorders, sexual dysfunction related to medical conditions, substance abuse dysfunctions, and psychological issues. Each of these can be traced to any of four common sources.

- **Brain health:** As we discussed in Part I, unbalanced brain chemistry can contribute to disorders of desire, arousal, orgasm, and/or sexual pain.

- **Hormonal health:** The loss of testosterone and other important hormones discussed in Chapter 9 can lead to a loss of libido (desire disorders) and difficulty achieving arousal and orgasm.

- **Overall physical health:** When your brain chemistry is compromised, so is your health, leading to a vast array of medical conditions that can affect your sex life. You'll learn more about this in Chapter 11, but it's important to recognize that 20 percent of men with ED also have diabetes; 12 percent also have a condition associated with heart disease.

ED Means DEAD Health

If your sexual function is not up to par, you may be physically ill. Here's why.

- Sexual function involves multiple organs and systems: vascular, neurological, and hormonal. If you are suffering from ED, at least one of these systems isn't working properly.
- ED is associated with cardiovascular disease: It is a marker of cardiovascular complications of high blood pressure.
- Low testosterone is associated with metabolic syndrome and type 2 diabetes.
- ED is a predictor of metabolic syndrome.
- Treatment of obesity improves sexual function.
- Treatment of depression improves ED.

- **Circulatory health:** When your brain is balanced, and you've addressed your hormones with bioidentical supplements, you may still have trouble with sexual performance. The issue might lie in your vasculature: your circulatory system. Forty-five percent of men with ED have high blood pressure, or hypertension.

Hypertension and GABA

Hypertension may be linked to excessive use of common pain relievers. Pain and emotional distress are certainly age accelerators that can lead to high blood pressure. And GABA deficiencies can lead to pain and anxiety that contribute to high blood pressure. Stresses ranging from retirement to marital problems have all been associated with high rates of stroke, even in nonhypertensive patients. So if you can boost your GABA, you'll see your blood pressure drop.

HEALTHY VASCULATURE LETS YOU KEEP IT UP LONGER

The vascular system carries the oxygen-rich blood away from the heart through blood vessels, arteries, and tiny capillaries, and returns it to the heart through the veins. Your blood pressure is such an important measurement of health because it determines how hard your heart has to work in order to circulate blood through your body.

As we age, the diameter of blood vessels can narrow and the arterial walls can stiffen from plaque buildup, which makes your heart work harder to move the same amount of blood through the body. This is what high blood pressure, a.k.a. hypertension, is all about. Even if your heart is functioning perfectly well, your vascular system can still be old.

Luckily (or unluckily) for men, the penis works like a vascular barometer. Your ability to obtain a strong erection is an indication that your vascular system is in good shape. Having a weak penis, or erectile dysfunction, could be an indication that your circulation is compromised. The *New York Times* reported that erectile problems may show up as early as

3 years before a cardiovascular event such as a heart attack or stroke. It only takes a small change in the penile artery to predict heart disease. By the time a man has erectile dysfunction, he's already pretty sick.

While this chapter focuses on that one important organ, it's also critical that you follow up on your overall health. A circulatory system malfunction, including an elevation in your blood pressure, can lead to a heart attack, stroke, and death.

High blood pressure is painless, symptomless, and often unexpected, although there is a genetic component. Though it is widely known that stress, tension, and nervousness cause hypertension, a calm and relaxed person can still have high blood pressure. It predominantly affects middle aged and elderly men, especially if they are obese or heavy drinkers. Most surprising is that 10 million of these victims are taking medications that are either of questionable value or may even be exacerbating their illness, and certainly negatively affecting their sexual performance.

BLOOD TEST	CHECKS FOR
Aldosterone and renin	Hormones produced by the adrenal glands that are elevated during high blood pressure
Antiphospholipid antibody	Increased risk for blood clots in arteries and veins
Factor V Leiden	Presence causes a lifelong risk for venous thrombosis
Fibrinogen	Abnormal levels linked with thrombosis or bleeding
Homocysteine	Elevated levels cause increased risk of venous and arterial thrombosis
Plasminogen	Decreased levels found in patients with venous thrombosis
Protein C and S; AT III	Deficiency causes increased risk for thromboembolism
Prothrombin	Mutation in prothrombin gene, which causes increased risk of venous thrombosis
Urine microalbumin	The presence of albumin in the urine, which could be an indication of high blood pressure

Blood Tests Monitor Peripheral Vascular Problems

The blood tests listed above can let you know if your vascular barometer is working. Your penis might be signaling a bigger problem than ED.

How Erectile Dysfunction Fits In

These same changes in blood flow are a major reason that the brain shrinks and sexual desire lessens as we age. The peripheral vascular system contains the smallest blood vessels and capillaries traveling to all of your appendages, including your penis. If these appendages aren't getting enough blood, or are getting the right amount of blood but aren't getting it fast enough, you're going to notice cold hands, cold feet, and a limp playmate.

When we are sexually aroused, the brain sends a nerve impulse in the form of the chemical nitric oxide, which is released in the endothelial cells of the blood vessels, telling the smooth muscles in the arteries of the penis to widen and relax, allowing blood to flow into the two cylindrical, spongelike structures called the corpus cavernosa. These tubes run along the length of the penis, parallel to the urethra, the tube that carries semen and urine. The sudden influx of blood expands the corpus cavernosa and produces an erection by straightening and stiffening the penis. Continued sexual arousal maintains the higher rate of blood flow into the penis and limits the blood flow out of the penis, keeping the penis firm.

But when the peripheral vascular system

is compromised, the penis won't work properly. Either the nitric oxide message gets lost or cannot be carried out. These issues prevent blood from flowing to the penis, which limits your ability to achieve or maintain an erection. Blood flow issues can result from hypertension, high cholesterol, vascular disease, diabetes, toxic exposure, drug abuse, smoking, and more. There can also be a structural deformity of the pudendal artery, which prevents blood flow as well.

Keeping the blood flowing to your brain is just as important as keeping the blood flowing to your penis. Decreased blood flow toward your brain diminishes brain function, which in turn reduces your sexual function. If you can increase blood flow in both directions through medications, hormones, nutrients, diet, and even exercise, you will be able to improve sexual function and reverse aging.

How Viagra Works

Viagra, Levitra, and Cialis are all phosphodiesterase inhibitors (known as PDE-5 inhibitors) that can treat the symptoms of ED by improving arterial blood flow. They work because they all promote the release of nitric oxide. However, it's important to recognize that these medications don't produce a spontaneous erection or increase your libido. They are not aphrodisiacs, so they will not work in the absence of sexual desire. Instead they allow an erection to occur after the desire and arousal states have been achieved. For most users, these drugs take at least 30 minutes or so to work, and you have a 4- to 24-hour window of opportunity, depending on which medication you choose. The results are exactly what you've heard, which is why these medications are often overused or incorrectly prescribed.

There are also serious side effects to consider. They can cause backaches, upset stomach, headaches, hearing loss, nasal congestion, and impaired vision. These medications can be taken with food (but not grapefruit juice; you're going to have to give up that morning beverage), and it is recommended that you avoid alcohol, as drinking may increase the likelihood of some side effects. Not all men can or should take them, especially if you have severe heart disease or heart failure, have had a stroke, have very low blood pressure, or have uncontrolled high blood pressure (hypertension), arrhythmias, or diabetes. Viagra, Levitra, and Cialis are not a good choice for you if you are currently taking:

Painful Erections

Painful or decreased fullness of erection might be related to vascular disease (in which case Viagra might work for you) or other medical disorders (where it may not be so effective). Another cause can be your own tension. Like painful constipation, you might inadvertently be holding ejaculate to the point of pain because you are too tense to let go.

Viagra Won't Help if You Suffer From:

- Brain chemical imbalances
- Chronic anxiety
- Low hormone levels
- Medical conditions that contribute to sexual dysfunction
- Neuropathy, or damaged nerves

- Nitrate drugs such as nitroglycerin (Nitro-Bid and others), isosorbide mono-nitrate (Imdur), or isosorbide dinitrate (Isordil)
- Blood-thinning (anticoagulant) medication
- Certain types of alpha blockers for enlarged prostate or high blood pressure

Not only are these drugs not a cure for circulatory problems, but they aren't even a cure for erectile dysfunction: They are simply a treatment for a symptom. I find it very interesting that the refill rate for these drugs is less than 50 percent: That means that while lots of men try them, these drugs often don't meet their expectations. As you've learned, sexual arousal issues can be caused by many things, including an imbalance in your brain chemistry. Sometimes, when the underlying issue is addressed or resolved, the need for Viagra and medications like it diminishes. In other cases, the erectile dysfunction issues may be permanent, requiring long-term usage of these medications.

Check Your Penile Blood Pressure

Your doctor will need to examine you before he recommends any prescription medication. He will likely require a physical evaluation to assess possible nerve damage and see if you have normal touch sensation in your genital area. Others tests that can be performed include:

- **Penile brachial pressure index (PBPI)** is a screening test that involves the measurement of penile and arm blood pressure.
- **Penile Doppler ultrasound** detects physical impediments to blood flow within the penis. The penis is injected

Penis Problems

Peyronie's disease is a connective tissue disorder involving the growth of fibrous plaque in the soft tissue of the penis, which affects 1 to 4 percent of men. Also known as bent nail syndrome, it causes the penis to become misshapen when erect, as well as causes painful erections. The hardened scar tissue known as plaques can cause a curvature of the penis or indentations. The condition may also make sexual intercourse painful and/or difficult, yet many men report satisfactory intercourse despite the disease. Peyronie's disease is not contagious, nor is it related to cancer. Treatment is available as either oral or injected anti-inflammatories such as para aminobenzoate potassium (Potaba), vitamin E therapy, or surgery. Another option is to inject a drug into the plaque to dissolve it.

with a medication that causes an erection. The blood flow to the penis at the time of erection is measured with an ultrasound wand to determine the degree of vascular abnormality. The entire procedure takes about 30 minutes to complete and is extremely precise.

- **Dynamic infusion cavernosometry and cavernosography (DICC)** involves injecting a vasodilator and dye into penile blood vessels followed by an x-ray in order to view abnormalities in blood pressure and blood flow into and out of your penis.

- **Biopsy of penile tissue** tests for the presence of nitric oxide, which is correlated with the integrity of penile nerves.

DRUGS THAT MAKE A DIFFERENCE

If you do have a vascular problem and erectile dysfunction, medications like Levitra, Cialis, and Viagra can be helpful. Papaverine and phentolamine are two other choices worth considering. They belong to the group of medicines called vasodilators, which are used to cause blood vessels to expand, thereby increasing blood flow. They are injectable medications that are used to produce erections. They are also used as part of a three-drug combination of papaverine, phentolamine, and alprostadil (a synthetic version of the hormone prostaglandin) to treat erectile dysfunction.

Many antihypertension drugs that do treat circulatory issues are well known to contribute to sexual dysfunction. However, the active ingredient in Cozaar and Hyzaar can significantly improve the sex lives of men as well as treat their overall vasculature. According to a report released by Wake Forest University Baptist Medical Center, sexual dysfunction in men with high blood pressure was aided by Cozaar.

CONVENTIONAL TREATMENT	DOSAGE
Cialis	10–20 mg per day before sexual activity or 2.5 mg once daily regardless of sexual activity
Cozaar	25–100 mg per day
Hyzaar	50/12.5–100/25 mg per day
Levitra	5–20 mg per day 1 hour before sexual activity
Papaverine	30–60 mg injected into base of penis per day up to 3 times per week and no more than 2 days in a row
Phentolamine	0.5–1 mg injected into the penis per day up to 3 times per week and no more than 2 days in a row
Viagra	25–100 mg per day 1 hour before sexual activity

In a group of hypertensive men treated with Cozaar, 88 percent reported improvement in at least one area of sexual dysfunction after 12 weeks of treatment.

NUTRIENTS CAN SUPPORT MAXIMUM SEXUAL PERFORMANCE

Before you rush to take Viagra-like medications, you should try to resolve erectile dysfunction through safer but equally effective nutrient programs. There are many nutrients that have been identified to keep blood moving efficiently through your brain, body, and penis. Look to the following to support your circulatory health.

- **Fish oils** improve blood flow.
- **French maritime pine bark** activates nitric oxide.
- **Icariin** is a natural plant extract used in traditional Chinese medicine. It has

Don't Use Sex to Mask a Deeper Issue

Don Juan is not just a famous fictional character: The name has been given to a real psychological condition that causes men to act as if they have an extremely high sex style in all areas of brain chemistry. However, they may be pursuing sexual activities compulsively in an attempt to mask deeper feelings of inferiority. It may also be an attempt to mask homosexual thoughts or feelings. However, studies show that as many as 20 percent of all people—men and women—experience a same-sex fantasy or thought sometime in their lives. It doesn't mean that you have a deep-seated sexual preference.

been shown to deactivate the enzyme normally responsible for winding down male sexual response, further promoting sustained activity. Scientists have noted that it acts like testosterone. However, if you have diabetes and/or significant kidney or liver disease, please consult with your health care practitioner before using this product.

- **L-arginine** is the biological precursor to nitric oxide synthesis in the endothelium. Arginine may be helpful for improving circulation to the penis. High doses of arginine have been shown to enhance sexual arousal, satisfaction, and performance.
- **Tribulus terrestris** is an herb that has been used in both China and India for centuries and is thought to increase sexual stamina, desire, and performance in men. It may also stimulate sperm as well as semen production. This herb may have the ability to increase the body's production of luteinizing hormone, which stimulates testosterone production. It may also help the conversion of androstenedione to testosterone.
- **Vitamin E** improves blood flow.

Fruits, Herbs, and Spices to Increase Circulation

- **Butcher's broom** may improve blood circulation.
- **Cayenne** may improve blood circulation because of its primary nutrient, capsaicin.

Pomegranate Perks You Up

Pomegranate fruits, juices, and extracts are thought to improve blood flow through all of your vasculature, but buyers beware. Pomegranate juice and extracts are expensive. Choose 100 percent pure juice whenever possible, or at least the highest concentration of juice available. Avoid "fruit cocktails" as they contain large amounts of sugary fructose.

- **Celery seeds** may improve blood circulation.
- **Cinnamon** increases circulation, especially in arthritic joints.
- **Cocoa** may improve blood circulation.
- **Garlic** aids in circulation and lowers blood pressure.
- **Ginger** enhances circulation.
- **Ginkgo biloba** may improve blood circulation.
- **Grapes** (purple and red) may improve the ability of the endothelium of blood vessels to dilate, which improves blood circulation.
- **Hawthorn** may improve blood circulation by dilating the blood vessels.
- **Onion** controls inflammation and aids in blood flow.
- **Schisandra** may improve blood circulation.
- **Siberian ginseng** may improve blood circulation.
- **Turmeric** increases blood flow.

PRELOX PUTS IT ALL TOGETHER

Many of the best sex-enhancing nutrients, including arginine, French maritime pine bark, and icariin, work better together than they do independently. For example, Prelox Natural Sex for Men has yielded compelling and highly satisfactory results in my office as well as five independent clinical studies. I'm so impressed that I recommend it to all my ED patients, certainly before I have them take prescription medications.

Prelox features Pycnogenol, a particular pine bark extract that has been shown to stimulate endothelial nitric oxide production from the arginine compound instead of the blood vessels, so that you can maintain an erection. The icariin acts to block phosphodiesterase-5, an enzyme that causes erections to subside. Working together, these nutrients not only promote harder, longer-lasting erections, but they can also increase fertility and augment endothelial health. What's more, many studies are showing that this compound may be more effective than Viagra, which only blocks the action of phosphodiesterase-5 without creating additional nitric oxide.

The five independent studies show that not only was sexual function restored, but they also point to an increase in the study participants' SexQ. For example, participants

Supplements Are Not All the Same

When it comes to supplements, always go with a name you trust: Many unscrupulous supplement manufacturers spike herbal preparations with the same prescription vasodilators found in Viagra, Cialis, and Levitra. Unlike other performance enhancement supplements marketed as "natural," Prelox Natural Sex for Men is not adulterated with trace amounts of prescription drugs.

reported that they had an increase in sexual dreams and fantasies and more frequent morning erections. Their partners noted higher sexual interest and enhanced sexual performance. This means that Prelox was able to reset the brain and enhance the users' SexQ, particularly by increasing acetylcholine, which is related to nitric oxide. More than 60 percent of the men in the studies reported that when they used Prelox it was easier to initiate erections and sustain them, and overall sexual experience was enhanced.

Better still, by improving endothelial health, you are also treating the larger issues related to overall circulation. Endothelial dysfunction leads to constriction of blood vessels, inflammation, and increased blood clotting. By increasing nitric oxide, you are also preventing these symptoms, along with cardiovascular disease.

WHEN SURGERY IS REQUIRED

Surgical techniques used for treating ED have not always yielded satisfying results. One common outcome is a shortened penis. However, if you have severe erectile dysfunction, you may want to talk with your physician about penile implants and other forms of surgery.

Inflatable penile implants are often used to replace the corpus cavernosa. This technique is performed primarily as a therapeutic surgery for men suffering from complete impotence. The implanted pump, which is placed near the scrotum, can be manipulated by hand to fill these cylinders from an implanted reservoir in order to achieve an erection. The replacement cylinders are normally sized to be direct replacements for the corpus cavernosa, but larger ones can be implanted. One advantage to this surgery is

Men Need Candy

At least nuts and chocolate. All types of tree nuts are high in L-arginine, which can enhance erectile performance. Chocolate is packed with epicatechins, the plant flavonoids that benefit your blood vessels.

Choose foods that are the building blocks of acetylcholine, listed in Chapter 5: They will enhance nitric oxide production. However, choose wisely: Too much fat will block nitric oxide (NO) production. You'll also want to avoid foods that block acetylcholine, including those in the nightshade family: white potatoes, green and red peppers, eggplant, tomatoes, and paprika.

Be Careful What You Wish For

Priapism is a prolonged, involuntary erection that is painful, is not associated with sexual stimulation, and can result in impotence. It is caused by inflow of blood to the penis in excess of outflow. It can occur from an imbalance in brain chemistry or as a side effect of certain medications or alcohol abuse. It is a common myth that men taking Viagra will be able to achieve long-standing erections, but I can assure you that it's not something to look forward to.

that an erection can be created whenever desired, for as long and as firm as desired.

Semirigid devices have an outer shell with a central core of metal or plastic. These prostheses are implanted and produce constant penile rigidity. The primary advantage of these devices is their ease of implantation. The disadvantages include a constantly rigid penis that does not look like a normal erection or one in a state of flaccidity.

Penile artery bypass surgery, or penile revascularization, may offer a permanent cure and allow men with ED to reverse this disease and return to spontaneously developing erections. The procedure is able to increase the erection blood flow. However, in a broad-spectrum survey of ED patients, only 2 to 3 percent meet the criteria for penile revascularization, which requires true artery blockage as compared to vascular pathology.

TOYS WORTH TRYING: A CES DEVICE

Cranial electrical stimulation, or CES, is a therapeutic tool that uses mild electronic stimulation to treat sexual dysfunction as well as anxiety, depression, and insomnia. CES alters the abnormal electrical connections and normalizes dysfunctional brain patterns that can be caused by environmental toxins, electromagnetic frequency (too much cell phone exposure), or brain chemistry imbalances. In short, CES helps balance your brain waves and your brain chemistry. It has been shown to raise the level of conversion of amino acids into dopamine and to increase blood levels of endorphins, which influence the ability for sexual desire, arousal, and response. It promotes the conversion of choline to produce acetylcholine and can improve GABA by relaxing the user so that he or she feels less overwhelmed. Lastly, by addressing insomnia, the device can improve serotonin levels.

Obtaining a CES device requires a prescription from a physician. I have been prescribing the CES device to my patients for more than 15 years and have seen hundreds of positive responses. The CES device is particularly effective for men who are prone to tension or who have had issues with substance abuse.

Positive results may be experienced immediately, though for some, it takes up

Sex Could Be Better if You're Not on Top

You don't have to control everything about sex in order to get what you want. Point of fact: Too much thrusting can weaken your erection, especially if you already know that you have heart disease or vascular disorders. The fix is simple: Lie on your back and let your partner do the work.

to 3 or 4 weeks. You can use a CES device for 45 minutes every evening while relaxing, reading, or watching TV.

Most people don't realize that when they touch each other, electric current passes through their bodies. We demonstrate this in my office by having couples practice touch with a CES device attached to their wrists. When they touch each other's hands and each other's breasts and head, they can feel current passing from one to the other. Or, when they touch themselves, they can feel current running through their nipples, clitoris, or penis. This exercise helps them understand the power of touch.

A LAST WORD TO THE WISE: PROTECT YOURSELF FROM SEXUALLY TRANSMITTED DISEASES

People with a high dopamine or a high serotonin SexQ love to experiment with lots of partners. The Centers for Disease Control recently released new numbers on STDs,

and there were nearly 19 million new sexually transmitted disease infections in 2008.

In case you forgot the list, here's what you could be in for.

- Chlamydia
- Genital warts
- Gonorrhea
- Hepatitis
- Herpes
- HIV
- Syphilis

Infections related to chlamydia and gonorrhea can cause epididymitis, a painful infection in the tissue surrounding the testicles. In addition, chlamydia may cause urethritis. Studies also suggest that the presence of a chlamydia or gonorrhea infection can increase your risk of HIV. The majority of reported syphilis cases are among men who have sex with men.

Most STDs can be well treated if you catch them at early stages. So again, if you see something, say something, and let your doctor know where you've been.

STD Tests: Early Detection Is Key

TEST	DISEASE
FTA-ABS, TPPA, Darkfield Microscopy, RPR, VDRL, EIA	Syphilis
Hep A, B, C, D, E	Hepatitis
Chlamydia Ab, urine	Chlamydia
Herpes I, II IGM, IGG, and 6 Abs	Herpes virus

PART IV

Younger and Healthier Is Sexier

CHAPTER 11

Old Body, Old Sex

YOUR SEXUALITY IS a marker of your overall health. When your interest in sex, as well as your performance level, is high, I can guarantee that you won't be complaining of any health problems. But when your sex life begins to lag, don't dismiss it by thinking your life is becoming too complicated, too tiring, or too busy. It's a clear sign that some aspect of your health is failing.

Sexual dysfunction can be secondary to a myriad of diseases and conditions. Many medical conditions can make you older by draining your hormone levels. What's more, when the problem begins with an aging sexuality, your overall health can topple like a row of dominoes. This is how both men and women react without the proper levels of sex hormones.

Heart: The heart's ability to pump blood, your peripheral vascular system, and the amount of blood getting to your brain are all dependent on your levels of estrogen, progesterone, and testosterone. And as sex hormones decrease, cholesterol increases.

Immune system: Sex hormones keep your immune system from going wild. If these hormones get out of whack, your immune system will begin to shut down. And a decline in sex hormones results in a drop in glucagon, and blood sugar control is compromised. This results in an increase in inflammation, oxidation, dehydration, and calcification.

Bones: Each of the sex hormones perpetuates both parathyroid and growth hormone production, which maintains your bone density. When these hormones are out of balance, your bone density decreases.

Skin: Sex hormones keep your skin looking and feeling young. Some of the most recent cosmeceutical advances include creams containing natural estrogen supplements for the face to make skin firmer and looking younger.

Brain: Sex hormones affect your memory and attention. Testosterone helps your visual memory, and estrogen affects your attention, concentration, and working memory.

Tell Someone When You Don't Feel Like Having Sex

Talk to your doctor about chronic medical conditions and their associated issues with sexual arousal or performance. More importantly, talk with your spouse/partner. If your health is holding you back, small changes, like timing medication differently or trying new sexual positions, may alleviate much of your discomfort during sex.

Because of these direct connections between sex and general well-being and youthful vitality, it is important to take care of your whole body so you can repair and reverse damage and get your sex life back on track.

THE PAUSES

Much as menopause and andropause mark a decline in hormone production, the rest of your internal organs age when they start to malfunction. I refer to these failing organs as experiencing pauses: time markers that identify the wear and tear of every part of the body. Like menopause, all of the pauses occur along with diminishing hormonal production, although sometimes they are not related to the sexual hormones.

During these pauses, the failing organ, or part, becomes older than the rest of your body and slowly, or in some cases rapidly, starts to die. When this occurs, its associated hormone levels drop, sending a signal to the rest of the body: Its purpose is to broadcast that the system is failing. This signal also begins the process whereby the whole body will begin to shut down. The following table shows each of the pauses and how they affect your sexuality as you age.

PAUSE	DECLINE IN	TYPICAL ONSET AGE	ASSOCIATED DISEASES THAT AFFECT SEX	HOW IT AFFECTS SEX
Adrenopause	DHEA	55	Adrenal disease	Decreased libido for men and women
Andropause	Testosterone in men	45	Prostate condition	Decreased libido for men
Dopamine biopause	Dopamine brain chemistry	30	Obesity and fatigue	Decreased libido for men and women
Acetylcholine biopause	Acetylcholine brain chemistry	40	Attention disorder and memory	Vaginal dryness for women, decreased arousal for men and women
GABA biopause	GABA brain chemistry	50	Anxiety, chronic pain, and sleep disorder	Decreased ability to achieve orgasm for men and women
Serotonin biopause	Serotonin brain chemistry	60	Depression and sleep disorder	Premature ejaculation for men, delayed orgasm for women

PAUSE	DECLINE IN	TYPICAL ONSET AGE	ASSOCIATED DISEASES THAT AFFECT SEX	HOW IT AFFECTS SEX
Cardiopause/ Vasculopause	Ejection fraction and blood flow	40	Cerebrovascular disease, circulatory system issues, coronary artery disease, hypertension	Decreased blood flow to genitals/erectile dysfunction for men, vaginal dryness for women, decreased sensation, arousal, and dyspareunia for both men and women
Dermatopause	Collagen, vitamin D synthesis	35	Scleroderma and loss of collagen; increased wrinkles	Skin conditions make sex uncomfortable
Immunopause	Hormonal and cellular immunity, T helper/ T suppressor ratio	40	Bacterial and viral infections and parasitic diseases	Painful intercourse
Insulopause	Glucose tolerance	40	Diabetes, neuropathy, and increase in body fat composition	Loss of sexual sensation, erectile dysfunction
Menopause	Estrogen, progesterone, and testosterone in women	40	All symptoms associated with menopause	Decrease in libido, arousal, lubrication, and orgasm
Sensory Pause	Touch, hearing, vision, and smell sensitivity	40	Decreased ability of all senses	Decreased arousal for men and women
Somatopause	Growth hormone	30	Increased body fat especially around the waist; anxiety and depression, fatigue, loss of muscle mass, reduced strength and stamina, and reduced bone density	Decreased libido for men and women
Thyropause	Thyroid and calcitonin hormone levels	50	For thyroid: hyperthyroidism, hypothyroidism, weight gain, fatigue, depression, attention and memory problems, constipation, and hair loss For calcitonin: reduced bone density/weak bones	Decreased libido for men and women
Uropause	Bladder control	45	Urinary tract infections, urinary frequency, urgency, urinating in the middle of the night, incontinence, stress incontinence in women when they cough or sneeze, and post-void dribble in men	Creates anxiety and uncomfortable sex

Reverse the Pauses for Better Sex

In my book *Younger You,* I explore many of these same diseases and health conditions in much greater detail. The key to preventing illness is to detect a problem before it affects the rest of your body. The book includes a simple test you can take to identify which pauses you may be experiencing. This test is also available on my Web site, www.pathmed.com.

Many of these symptoms and conditions can be reversed by following the right treatment protocols, including prescription medications, proper diet, and nutritional supplementation. Good health in every area of the body improves overall health. For example, when I fix someone's osteoporosis with parathyroid hormone, I balance it with testosterone, so their sex life improves along with their bone density. By fixing one pause, I actually fix two, and the effect is synergistic.

The overall goal with antiaging medicine is to keep you in the same vibrant health you have, or had, at age 40. By addressing the pauses, not only will you feel better, but you can increase your vitality and your physical strength, and reduce the likelihood of losing memory and attention. When you fix your sex life, your health gets better. If you fix your health, your sex life gets better.

The following are the areas of health that most directly affect sexual function. If you can circumvent their associated diseases, not only will you be able to add 15 good years to your life span, but you will be able to extend your sex life as well. That is sure to make you feel both younger and sexier.

METABOLIC SYNDROME: WHEN YOUR WAIST KILLS YOUR SEX LIFE

Forty percent of Americans over 40 have three or more of the following symptoms: abdominal obesity, increased triglycerides, dyslipidemia (low HDL cholesterol), hypertension, and hyperglycemia (elevated blood glucose). When these symptoms occur together, it is referred to as metabolic syndrome. All of these will affect your waist and your sexual performance: Obesity, for one, affects your heart muscles and blood flow, making sex (which should be quite vigorous!) much more difficult. To get your sex life back, you need to lose weight by losing body fat and gaining muscle, get your blood sugar stable, and reverse the damage done.

THE PROBLEM WITH DIABETES

An estimated 18.2 million Americans have diabetes, and it is assumed that almost one-third have no idea that they have this disease. Diabetes occurs when the body can no longer correctly process the sugars it takes in from carbohydrate-dense foods like white rice, white flour, and potatoes. The body should be able to break down these foods into simple sugars, or glucose, and use this by-product for cellular fuel. The hormone insulin should transport the glucose to the cells. However, when the body does not produce enough insulin, the glucose just sits there, building up in the bloodstream, causing a condition called hyperglycemia, or high blood sugar. This condition sets up a cascade of events that contribute to inflammation and plaque deposition within the vascular system and high blood pressure. Conversely, high blood pressure and other vasculopause conditions can contribute to diabetes. If this condition has been with you since birth, you suffer from type 1 diabetes. However, if you have developed this later in life, you are likely suffering from type 2 diabetes.

Diabetes is closely linked to obesity. Excess weight caused by the overconsumption of carbohydrate-rich foods creates the initial insulin resistance. A sedentary lifestyle also accounts for much of the diabetes epidemic. However, type 2 diabetes is completely preventable. The old diet routine—eat less, exercise more—is the prescription.

Men and women with diabetes often tell me that they are having difficulty with orgasm and sexual responsiveness. Blood sugar has actually damaged the nerve endings in the penis or the vagina, which literally stunts the person's ability to feel. The sugar sticks like glue to the blood vessels, nerves,

and veins, and everything is damaged. Without these nerve endings, it is impossible to be sensual or in touch with your partner. From my point of view, one of the hardest conditions to restore is a diabetic penis.

Diabetes is easily confirmed by measuring your blood glucose levels. You may notice many of the following symptoms if you are suffering from type 2 diabetes.

- Blurred vision
- Excessive thirst
- Extreme hunger
- Frequent urination
- Increased fatigue
- Irritability
- Weight gain

Control Your Blood Sugar for More Intense Sex

By integrating supplements, diet, medication, and exercise, you will have the best chance of beating this disease. Hormone balance is critical for diabetes management: A hormone deficiency can decrease the effectiveness of insulin. Growth hormone can help diabetes patients because they have significant muscle wasting. Growth hormone also increases sensitivity to insulin. Testosterone supplementation for men reduces insulin resistance, raises "good" HDL, lowers blood pressure, and helps to reduce excess weight while building muscle. Balancing estrogen, progesterone, and testosterone in women also improves glucose control and may alleviate the tendency to gain weight.

Supplements can help normalize blood sugar. These include the following:

- **Bilberry fruit extract** provides antioxidant and circulatory support
- **Chromium** protects against fatal arrhythmias for people with diabetes
- **Cinnamon** contains procyanidins, which boost insulin's activity about twentyfold
- **Essential fatty acids** prevent insulin resistance
- **Fish oil and DHEA** improve insulin sensitivity and optimize blood lipids
- **Lipoic acid** supports healthy nerve function
- **Psyllium, guar gum, and bilberry leaf extract** slow glucose absorption and prevent blood sugar spikes

BUILD BETTER BONES AND MUSCLES TO HAVE BETTER SEX

As a rule, we feel achier as we get older. We have stiffer joints, low muscle mass, and weaker bones. But this isn't all you have to look forward to: Your sexuality will also be damaged when you lose muscle mass and bone density. Your muscles work like a secondary heart—it aids in keeping your blood pumping. Without the proper amount of muscle, the blood flow to your brain and your genitals will diminish. In fact, by the ages of 60 to 70, the speed at which blood flows through the body is diminished by as much as 50 percent.

Poor bone structure means frailty and calcium deposits throughout your body, which stiffen you in places where you don't really want to be stiff. People with osteoporosis have calcium deposits in their brains, joints, kidneys, gallbladders, and heart. And you don't have to wait until you get old: I see lots of young people who are osteoporotic, and they have all sorts of sexual problems.

In order to keep your sex life active, you need to start preparing for your eighties now so that you can continue to grow new muscle and bone. The best way to rebuild muscle and bone is through eating right, exercise, and bioidentical hormone replacement therapies. For example, one patient of mine takes Cymbalta (duloxetine) to help him build new brain cells, Forteo (teriparatide) to give him new bone, and growth hormone to give him more muscle mass. Through this treatment, he will become a younger, sexier, 67-year-old who can stay that way for another 15 years.

Forteo is a synthetic form of parathyroid hormone. This treatment can stimulate bone formation and growth, repair connective tissue, prevent calcification, and increase bone density. Forteo has been shown to significantly increase spinal bone density in postmenopausal women with osteoporosis. It may have the potential to reverse depleted bone stores as well as prevent further bone loss by stimulating an increase in bone mass and bone strength.

DIAGNOSTIC TESTS TO MEASURE BONE AND MUSCLE LOSS	NATURAL TREATMENTS	FOODS THAT BUILD BONES AND MUSCLES	HORMONAL TREATMENTS	CONVENTIONAL TREATMENTS
• Boron and strontium—low boron and strontium levels contribute to osteoporosis • Calcitonin—hormone involved with maintaining bones • Parathyroid hormone—maintains bones • Urine telopeptides—when you lose bone, you are also losing telopeptides that are excreted in urine • Vitamin D/Vitamin K—related to bone loss	• Black cohosh • Boron • Calcium • Copper • Ipriflavone • Magnesium • Manganese • Omega-3's • Omega-6's • Red clover • Silica • Soy isoflavonoids • Strontium • Vitamin C • Vitamin K_1 • Zinc	• Almonds • Brazil nuts • Broccoli • Cabbage • Cantaloupe • Cheese • Chickpeas • Collard greens • Eggs • Flaxseeds • Grapefruit • Grape seed oil • Guava • Kale • Lean beef • Legumes • Mackerel • Mangoes • Milk • Mustard greens • Oat bran • Olive oil • Oranges • Peppers • Pinto beans • Pistachio nuts • Red leaf lettuce • Safflower oil • Salmon • Sardines • Sesame seeds • Soy/tofu • Spinach • Strawberries • Sunflower oil • Tomatoes • Tuna • Turnip greens • Walnuts • Yogurt	• Calcitonin (Miacalcin) • Estrogen • Growth hormone • Parathyroid hormone (Forteo) • Progesterone • Testosterone • Vitamin D_2 • Vitamin D_3	• Actonel • Boniva • Fosamax

KEEP YOUR KIDNEYS CLEAR

Erectile dysfunction and impotence occur in close to 50 percent of patients who undergo dialysis. When the kidneys cannot function properly, they cannot help the body clear itself of other illnesses. The kidneys function as filters of drugs and toxins in the body. Advanced kidney disease can only be treated with dialysis or by kidney transplant.

Chronic kidney disease occurs as a result of damage to the filtering tubes in the kidneys, and is consequently marked by persistent proteinuria, or excessive protein in the urine. Many of these patients also have decreased testosterone levels, autonomic neuropathy, and accelerated vascular disease, and are taking multiple medications that can affect sexual function. The kidneys are half dead in most people by 50 years of age. This occurs where there is either obesity or vascular disease like high blood pressure, or both.

People with advancing kidney failures feel very ill, especially when they experience "toxic uremia." This occurs when nitrogen levels build up in your blood because the kidneys are no longer working efficiently. Nitrogen makes you feel ill all the time, and nobody feels sexy when they have nitrogen in their blood.

Growth hormone and the drug Increlex are being studied as possible new treatments because they can build muscle. However, prevention is the most effective mode of combating kidney failure. To prevent kidney failure:

- Avoid taking large amounts of over-the-counter medications, including aspirin, acetaminophen, and ibuprofen. Consult a doctor before taking these medications on a daily basis.
- Avoid consumption of alcohol, which can damage the kidneys.
- Don't use illegal drugs, including heroin, cocaine, and Ecstasy, which can cause high blood pressure, stroke, heart failure, and even death, in some cases from only one use. Cocaine, heroin, and amphetamines can cause kidney damage.

THE VERY BEST PHYSICAL IS A *STAR TREK* PHYSICAL

If you can detect illness at the earliest possible point, you can reverse disease and extend your sexuality. However, the problem often starts in the doctor's office. The American physical exam has not been updated for nearly 100 years. I know that a computer can do a better job than fingers and stethoscopes as long as doctors know what to do with the data, including working with radiologists who know how to identify all the lumps and bumps of the human body.

An ultrasound exam allows doctors to see the condition and function of every organ. We can see nodules, precancers, damage, change in shape and size due to disease or dysfunction, inflammation, calcifications, and dehydration. Physicians cannot possibly detect all of these irregularities in the course of a manual physical exam. And you pay the consequences when they miss: The disease grows, spreads, becomes more invasive, and begins to affect other areas of the body, or worse, leads to an early death.

The ultrasounds listed here form the backbone of the physical that should be employed to get the very best health care. MRIs, CAT scans, and PET scans are all effective for specific diseases, but nothing compares to the ultrasound in terms of its global general review.

- **Abdominal ultrasound** shows enlarged liver or spleen; shows early changes of alcoholic hepatitis, nonalcoholic fatty liver, gallstones, gallbladder wall thickening, liver cyst, hemangiomas, other benign tumors and cancer, calcifications, cysts/calcifications of pancreas, and enlargement or atherosclerotic changes in abdominal aorta. Can identify damage due to drugs and infections. Can detect pancreatic cancer or previously benign cysts, sarcomas, abdominal aortic aneurysms, and spleen calcification.

- **Breast ultrasound** is the best test for finding breast cysts, nodules, masses, calcifications, and dense breast tissue. Can detect cancers and precancers.

- **Carotid ultrasound** measures blood flow through the main artery in the neck to the brain. Can show early changes in blood flow, intimal thickening, or advanced atherosclerotic disease blockages.

- **Echocardiogram** shows heart size (all four chambers), ejection fraction, valvular disease, changes in wall motion as a sign of previous or current heart attack and/or heart failure, and early changes in heart appearance. Can predict early changes/enlargements in ventricles and atrium, atrial fibrillations, and coronary artery disease.

- **Pelvic ultrasound** shows uterine enlargement, fibroids, changes in ovaries (increased size, cysts, tumors), prominent endometrium, cervical cysts, sarcomas, and fluid collection due to advancing ovarian cancer. It can also identify bladder size and bladder stones.

- **Prostate ultrasound** shows size of prostate, its nodules, calcifications, mass, bladder size and function, or presence of residual urine in patient with enlarged prostate.

- **Renal ultrasound** shows kidney stones/

The Best Over-the-Counter Antiaging Therapies

- Acetyl-L-Carnitine: boosts memory and attention
- Aspirin: reduces inflammation
- Carnosine: powerful antioxidant
- Coenzyme Q10: may lower blood pressure and decrease migraines
- Fish oil: a good fat high in omega-3
- Folic acid, vitamin B_6, and vitamin B_{12}: mood stabilizer and sleep enhancer
- Green tea extract: increases metabolism and overall energy
- L-Alpha GPC (glycerylphosphorylcholine): enhances overall brain function
- Melatonin: improves ability for restful sleep
- Nexrutine and 5-Loxin: reduces chronic pain

cysts/tumors, fluid collection in kidneys (hydronephrosis), and enlargement or kidney atrophies.

- **Scrotal ultrasound** shows size of testicles and epididymis, presence of varicocele, spermatocele, water in testicles, changing size of testicles, calcifications, and tumors, and can diagnose infertility, cancer, and overuse of testosterone.
- **Thyroid ultrasound** shows changes to thyroid size, cancer, masses, nodules, calcifications, cysts, and atrophy for earliest possible diagnosis of disease.
- **Transcranial ultrasound** measures blood flow in the main arteries of the brain. It can detect aneurysms and damaged blood vessels, provide information regarding migraines and dementia, and also detect increased velocity of blood flow due to vascular spasm or blockage.

CHAPTER 12

A Younger (Sexier) You Is Thinner and More Fit

ONCE YOU BEGIN to get your health back on track by following the Younger (Sexier) You program, you'll likely experience vast changes to your SexQ. You might start to feel increased sexual desire, or even find that arousal and orgasms come easier. If you are supplementing with natural bioidentical hormones or nutrients, you may feel that sex is more comfortable, more enjoyable, and even more fun.

Don't stop there! You've taken some very important steps, but there's more work to be done. Now it's time to focus on how you look, not just how you feel. I want you to feel good about yourself, in and out of bed, and for most of us, that means taking off a few extra pounds. And while dieting might not be your thing, studies show that losing weight can result in significant improvements in sexual functioning and satisfaction. Those who exercise regularly have higher levels of desire and enhanced ability to be aroused and achieve orgasm. My office is restoring sexuality every day to my patients who lose weight. All of a sudden

they find themselves as sexually active as they were when they were 20 years old. So if you are overweight, losing between 8 and 20 pounds will help you look younger and feel sexier. And that's worth 7 to 10 more years of great sex, and a more intimate relationship with your partner.

THE SEESAW OF SEX AND APPETITE

Sex and food are central human appetites, so it's not hard to understand how both can become addictive. However, they seem to have an inverse relationship. When you're

The Most Desired Body

Both men and women find slimness attractive. In a study conducted at the University in Tübingen, Germany, the frequency of penile-vaginal intercourse was highest among participants who had a slimmer waist and slimmer hips. Another study puts more emphasis on whittling your middle: The body type that men currently prefer has a high waist to hip ratio, which is considered even more attractive than large breasts.

engaged in frequent and loving sexual relations, your appetite for food seems to diminish. However, when sexual appetite isn't satisfied, food cravings go up. In a Tübingen, Germany, study, slimness was negatively associated with frequency of masturbation for both sexes. The likely sexual scenario is that the majority of heavy people masturbate alone, while the slim ones are having sex with each other. Being overweight can be a signal to potential sexual partners that the soothing effects of overeating are more important to you than the pleasures of intercourse.

The goal is to master all your appetites, including your sexuality. Sex, like food, is another important tool that can help enhance all aspects of your life, including love, work, thinking, stability, and rest. Without a fully engaged sexual life, you may end up either losing your sexuality entirely or gorging yourself to obesity.

DIET FOR A YOUNGER (SEXIER) YOU

A healthy diet and active lifestyle are the keys to losing weight and staying fit. The food suggestions in Chapters 4, 5, 6, and 7 are meant to enhance specific brain chemicals that will increase your desire, arousal, ability to orgasm, and sexual resolution and are just one important part of the Younger (Sexier) You program. My book, *Younger (Thinner)*

You Diet, uses these same foods in combination with other tools in order to achieve lasting weight loss. It outlines how you can boost metabolism and choose nutrient-dense foods that will not only facilitate weight loss but improve brain function.

This same diet is perfect for upgrading your sex life, because dopamine controls both metabolism and your sexual fire. The same foods that will speed your metabolism will reignite the passion in your love life. The same acetylcholine foods will increase arousal as well as improve thinking, so you can make better decisions about the foods you eat. GABA foods keep you calm, so you won't fall into the trap of emotional eating, and orgasm can come more easily. Lastly, serotonin foods allow your brain to reboot, so your sexual timing will be improved and you can get a good night's rest.

Weight gain is a very common side effect of both menopause and andropause. By following the Younger (Thinner) You Diet, you'll be able to control your weight and stop the cascade of illness associated with obesity while increasing your hormone production. It's remarkable how carrying as few as 10 extra pounds can significantly affect your overall health.

However, it's important that you take a slow and steady approach to weight loss. When you reduce your intake of calories by more than 15 percent from what you are currently eating, your body is tricked into thinking it is starving and it reduces the production of testosterone, which is exactly what you don't want. A high metabolism, high dopamine diet is meant to increase testosterone, so you can increase your libido.

This chapter highlights the main concepts of the Younger (Thinner) You Diet, which allows you to choose from a wide variety of fresh foods, herbs, spices, and teas that will help you lose weight and keep those pounds from coming back. These foods have been specially chosen to create long-lasting satiety so you won't feel hungry.

Eating foods that are nutrient dense, rather than calorie dense, is the key to maintaining weight loss. You want every square inch of your food to be packed with nutrients, not calories. Low-volume, high-caloric foods can delay the brain and stomach's activation of the feeling of fullness, so you eat more of these poor food choices.

Rule #1: Spices Sex You Up for Weight Loss

Herbs and spices are an integral part of the Younger (Thinner) You Diet. Spices and herbs maximize nutrient density because they contain antioxidants, minerals, and multivitamins without a single additional calorie. Every time you add spice, you're adding nutrients and upgrading your meal.

Herbs and spices are just as important as fruits and vegetables for their antioxidant content and healing power. I tell all my patients to spice up every meal by adding three spices to each dish. You'll create super foods that are abundantly healthy and loaded with cancer-preventing properties.

The table on page 176 shows the antioxidant value of each herb and spice. ORAC stands for Oxygen Radical Absorbance Capacity, the method of measuring the antioxidant capacity of different foods developed by the National Institutes of Health. The higher values imply stronger antioxidant capabilities.

Mediocre foods, like plain whole wheat toast, can be upgraded into quality foods with a sprinkling of cinnamon. And because spices are nutrient dense, they are thermogenic, which means they naturally increase your metabolism.

Some spices and herbs increase your overall feeling of fullness and satiety too, so you'll eat less. One study, conducted at Maastricht University in the Netherlands, showed that when healthy subjects consumed an appetizer containing half a teaspoon of red-pepper flakes before each meal, it decreased their calorie intake by 10 to 16 percent. And when you flavor your foods with spices instead of salt, you'll immediately see the difference in your body, with less of the bloating and water retention caused by salty foods. Without salt in your diet, your overall health improves, especially if you have high blood pressure.

Total ORAC Values for Herbs and Spices*

HERB/SPICE	ORAC/100 G
Basil, fresh	4,805
Cardamom	2,764
Chives, raw	2,094
Cilantro, raw	5,141
Cinnamon, ground	267,536
Cloves, ground	314,446
Cumin seed	76,800
Curry powder	48,504
Dill weed, fresh	4,392
Garlic powder	6,665
Ginger, ground	28,811
Marjoram, fresh	27,297
Mustard seed, yellow	29,257
Oregano, fresh	13,970
Paprika	17,919
Parsley, dried	74,349
Parsley, raw	1,301
Pepper, black	27,618
Peppermint, fresh	13,978
Poppy seeds	481
Sage, fresh	32,004
Savory, fresh	9,465
Tarragon, fresh	15,542
Thyme, fresh	27,426
Turmeric, ground	159,277

* *Oxygen Radical Absorbance Capacity (ORAC) of Selected Foods—2007; Nutrient Data Laboratory, US Department of Agriculture (USDA)*

Fresh Herb Facts

- 1 teaspoon dried herbs = 1 tablespoon fresh herbs
- Add fresh herbs near the end of your cooking time for the most flavor and benefits.
- Refrigerate fresh herbs except for basil, which is best stored at room temperature.

Rule #2: Drink Tea with Every Meal to Flush Fat and Boost Metabolism

Tea is an integral weight-loss and antiaging tool. This is due mainly to the nutrients it contains, namely polyphenols, which have powerful antioxidant properties. Darker teas have the highest concentrations and offer higher antioxidant values.

Tea has absolutely no calories (if you don't add milk or sugar) and can stimulate digestion, cleanse the body, reduce inflammation, lower cholesterol, and give you lots of energy. These are all necessary for losing weight and improving your sex life.

Choose any type of tea that you prefer, including decaffeinated or herbal varieties. However, green tea has been the subject of the most scientific research. Green tea can increase metabolism, decrease appetite, and provide more energy for exercise. Green tea may also reduce the absorption of dietary fats by approximately 40 percent by blocking the production of digestive enzymes that facilitate the absorption of dietary fats. It can also help reduce fat by inhibiting the effects of insulin so that sugars are sent directly to the muscles for instant use, instead of being stored as body fat.

Beware the very popular bottled teas: Their antioxidant levels are 10 to 100 times lower than those in brewed tea, and many of them are full of sugar. Instead of drinking bottled tea, I brew my own and often combine two or three varieties to get the most color, and therefore the most benefit. For example, I brew a pot that makes 3 to 4 cups, and I combine red rooibos, blueberry, and green tea.

Rule #3: Yogurt Boosts Passion for Easier Arousal

Make sure to eat a single 8-ounce cup of low-fat yogurt every day. Yogurt is high in both calcium and protein, which together are known to raise metabolism and improve digestion. Yogurt also supports your immune system, reduces overall inflammation, and lowers your LDL or "bad" cholesterol. Best of all, yogurt may

Rooibos Tea: Pure Nutrients with a Sexy Red Color

This South African herbal tea is packed with vitamin C, with 50 percent more antioxidants than its caffeinated rival, green tea. For an added nutrient bonus, try a rooibos tea brewed with cinnamon.

help burn fat and promote weight loss. A University of Tennessee study in 2005 shows that dieters who ate three servings of yogurt a day lost 22 percent more weight and 61 percent more body fat than those who simply cut calories and didn't add calcium to their eating plan. Calcium is an important part of the eating plan because it reduces belly fat.

Rule #4: Choose Lean Proteins to Enhance Dopamine and Desire

Too much red meat may thwart your best weight-loss efforts, which is why this diet emphasizes fish and poultry for protein choices. You can eat fish and chicken every day and choose from other proteins in moderation, including lamb, pork, veal, turkey, Cornish hen, soy, eggs and egg whites, and low-fat dairy products such as fat-free or low-fat milk and, of course, yogurt.

Rule #5: Balanced Foods Are the Best Choice

I've given up on the US government's food pyramid and its heavy emphasis on carbohydrates. In my opinion it is a medical disaster. Instead, I classify foods in two categories: expanding foods and balanced foods. Expanding foods are those that have extreme effects on the body, causing a seemingly positive short-term effect (an

energy boost) while creating a nutritional disaster over time. Once you start to eat expanding foods, you may find yourself craving more of them to restore your energy. Simple carbohydrates, refined foods, and "white foods" are all expanding foods because they boost your energy in the short term but often create food cravings, dopamine deficiencies, and worse, food addictions. These are foods that can zap energy and attention and make us feel "flighty."

Foods in this category include:

- Foods filled with saturated fats
- Foods high in salt
- Foods high in sugar
- Foods made from white flour
- Fried foods
- All "white" pastas (wheat, rice, gluten free)
- Processed foods
- White bread
- White rice

Younger (Thinner) You foods are balanced foods. The body still needs carbohydrates and proteins to stay healthy, but instead of making bad food choices in the extreme range of these categories, you can choose a middle option. Moderate portions of lean meats, fish, and poultry are all in the range of balanced foods. So are whole grains like millet, brown rice, barley, corn, oats, quinoa, and buckwheat. These foods are absorbed slowly by the body, thus keeping glucose and insulin

Is There Such a Thing as a Good Carb?

Yes! The best carbs for hormone balance and overall health are those closest to nature: unrefined whole grains and fiber-rich vegetables and fruits.

low and providing long-lasting energy. They provide the unique ability to prevent the steep declines in blood sugar levels that give rise to fatigue, mood swings, and food cravings.

Rule #6: Fiber Keeps Your Body Clean Inside and Out

Diets that are low in fat and high in fiber may be the most effective combination that promotes weight loss. Fiber is like a scrub brush for your digestion, scouring your system until it is sparkling clean. It cleans out your colon, controls your blood sugar, pulls fat from your arteries, raises your "good" (HDL) cholesterol, and detoxifies your body, making your skin sparkle. What's more, it's bulky: Fiber fills you up so you eat less and feel full faster.

There are two types of fiber, soluble and insoluble. Soluble fiber is acted upon by the normal bacteria in your intestines. Good sources of soluble fiber include oats, beans, dried peas, fruits, vegetables, and legumes. Insoluble fiber is not digested by the body and increases intestinal transit. It also promotes regularity and softens stools. Wheat bran, whole grain products, and vegetables are good sources of insoluble fiber.

The American Dietetic Association recommends that a healthy diet should include 25 to 35 grams of fiber a day, including both soluble and insoluble fiber. However, most Americans consume only about half that amount. Check labels for fiber content in baked goods and choose breads, cereals, and pastas made from whole grains. Leafy greens, root vegetables, and beans and lentils are all good sources. Other recommended fiber-abundant foods are quinoa, millet, bulgur, buckwheat, seeds, and nuts. They are absorbed slowly by the body, thus keeping glucose and insulin low and providing long-lasting energy. They possess the unique ability to prevent the steep declines in blood sugar levels that give rise to fatigue, mood swings, and food cravings.

Rule #7: Drink Water throughout the Day to Stay Lubricated

Water continuously flushes your digestive system, moving food particles along at a rapid rate, which leads to weight loss. And, if you're busy drinking your 3 to 4 liters of water all day, you won't have the time or the desire to drink higher-calorie beverages like sodas or juices.

Drinking coffee and teas counts, especially those with deep colors for a greater nutritional punch.

Drinking plenty of water will make your metabolism more thermogenic, because water raises your dopamine levels. Another benefit is that if you drink water 30 minutes prior to a meal, it will actually fill you up so you will eat less. This is especially true for older individuals. Even better, a well-hydrated body is a well-lubricated body, making sex much more comfortable.

Rule #8: Create a Rainbow in Every Meal

Fruits and vegetables are probably the most advantageous foods that we can choose, mostly because of their colorfulness. These colors are actually packed with phytonutrients, plant-derived compounds that help us maintain health. These phytonutrients run the gamut from providing extra fiber, vitamins that can prevent heart disease, and of course, powerful antioxidants that boost your immune system.

To ensure a healthy diet, I tell my patients to eat every color of the rainbow. And eat as much as you want: No one ever suffers from eating too much broccoli!

- Red fruits, like tomatoes, watermelon, and pomegranate, contain lycopene, which can support your cardiovascular system to keep blood pumping to all of your organs, including your brain and your genitals.

- Orange and yellow fruits and vegetables contain carotenoids that can protect vision, so you can enjoy the visual pleasure of intimacy.
- Green foods have lutein, which may decrease your risk of cancers and help maintain strong muscles and bones, which can help keep sex active.
- Blue, violet, and purple plants contain resveratrol, which can help keep the urinary tract free from infection, making sex more comfortable.

Rule #9: Choose Quality Produce

Some people doubt the necessity of organic foods, but I can tell you that if organic fruits and vegetables are more expensive, it's for a good reason. Organic produce is grown without harmful pesticides. Today's fruits and vegetables have just a fraction of the nutrient content they had just 20 years ago, because heavy use of pesticides and chemical fertilizers has destroyed the soil.

When you are shopping for fresh fruits and vegetables, the best choice is local and organic. The second best choice is local and conventionally farmed, because the fruit will have ripened on the tree longer. Concentrate on eating the highest-quality food you can afford to buy, and you'll do wonders for your overall health, and your waistline.

Fruits and vegetables contain higher amounts of fiber when they are eaten raw than when they are cooked. Many of the

The USDA's Top 20 Antioxidant-Rich Foods (Based on ORAC Values)

FOOD ITEM	SERVING SIZE	TOTAL ANTIOXIDANT CAPACITY PER SERVING SIZE
Red beans	½ cup	13,727
Wild blueberries	1 cup	13,427
Red kidney beans	½ cup	13,259
Pinto beans	½ cup	11,864
Blueberries	1 cup	9,019
Cranberries (whole)	1 cup	8,983
Artichokes (hearts)	1 cup	7,904
Blackberries	1 cup	7,701
Prunes	½ cup	7,291
Raspberries	1 cup	6,058
Strawberries	1 cup	5,938
Red Delicious apple	1	5,900
Granny Smith apple	1	5,381
Pecans	1 ounce	5,095
Sweet cherries	1 cup	4,873
Black plum	1	4,844
Russet potato	1	4,649
Black beans	½ cup	4,181
Plum	1	4,118
Gala apple	1	3,903

important nutrients, vitamins, and enzymes (which may help with digestion) are destroyed or inactivated during cooking, then thrown out with the boiling water. For example, steaming broccoli on a stovetop can deplete its vitamin C content by as much as 34 percent, reports the *Journal of Food Science*.

Rule #10: Eat from Three Food Groups at Each Meal

Choose one protein, then a complex carbohydrate, and a healthy fat of a different color. At the same time, make each meal at least 70 percent plant-based and no more than 30 percent animal-based.

Obesity = Lousy Sex

Increasing body mass index is associated with decreasing testosterone levels, lower dopamine activity, and a decreased sexual drive. This is one instance when size is working against you. What's more, an obese physique can mask the size of your genitals, making men look smaller than they actually are.

MORE ON LEPTIN

As you've learned, one of the most important ways to stay younger and become sexier is to keep your hormone levels high. Your body uses hormones as chemical regulators and messengers, and keeping them at optimal levels means your body is communicating well. This in turn leads to a healthy metabolism, which burns your food efficiently without gaining weight, as well as a highly active SexQ.

Leptin, as we discussed in Chapter 4, is a hormone secreted by your body's fat tissue. Leptin comes from the Greek word *leptos,* meaning "thin," and was so named because it tells the body to stop eating. The more leptin present, the less hungry we are. Leptin is connected to dopamine because when leptin is released, dopamine production also increases, so we feel satisfied sooner and eat less.

The recent discovery of this hormone has given doctors a better understanding of fat cells (adipocytes). These cells are no longer viewed as a part of tissue that merely stores excess calories. Instead, we now know that they are dynamic cells that work with the endocrine system to produce hormones that regulate your appetite and metabolism.

Leptin works in conjunction with two other hormones, proopiomelanocortin (POMC) and neuropeptide Y (NPY). These regulate appetite and body weight. Neurons that produce these hormones often have the majority of leptin receptors. NPY stimulates appetite, while POMC suppresses it. Hormonal imbalance, including leptin resistance, will lead to an increased NPY level, decreased POMC, and increased appetite. Boosting leptin and creating the right proportion of hormones decreases NPY and increases POMC, lessening appetite and enhancing metabolism.

The following foods should be incorporated into your meal plan every day because they stimulate leptin production. But if you were to choose just one, go for broccoli: It's high in fiber and contains leptin enhancers; it is also the best dopamine-enhancing food. So eat as much broccoli as you can, steamed, roasted, or raw.

- Apples
- Broccoli
- Carrots
- Egg whites
- Pomegranate juice
- Salmon
- Spinach
- Unsalted almonds

Obesity can also be traced to hidden illnesses: It can be a result of any type of brain chemical imbalance, medications, or disease.

You may find that once you balance your brain chemistry, your leptin will self-regulate to lower, or more stable, levels.

MORE HORMONES WORTH MONITORING

The hormone incretin is made in the gut and released in response to food. It enhances insulin production and decreases glucagon release, so that the carbohydrates you eat are used and not stored. It also helps the body process food by stimulating the pancreas to produce insulin. It inhibits gastric emptying and reduces appetite and food intake. When incretin levels are low, you feel hungry and gain weight. You can enhance your incretin level by taking a natural, bioidentical version, which you can obtain with a doctor's prescription.

Stress causes severe hormone imbalance, which can lead to decreased metabolism and weight gain. Any type of stress can increase your cortisol levels. Increased cortisol levels lead to increased leptin resistance, which contributes to even more weight gain. What's more, cortisol is also linked to increased belly fat. When excess cortisol is released, you get puffy everywhere, you can feel restless, and your appetite increases.

ANTI-NUTRIENTS ARE ANTI-SEX

Foods that make you gain weight are not only addictive but bad for your waist and bad for sex. They contribute to the breakdown of your body's metabolic machinery, which drains the brain of energy and sexual desire. The worst offenders are sugars, fats, and white flour.

You may be addicted to sugar if you crave something sweet—like a small bite of chocolate—after every meal, or if you think about dessert all day. With the American adult obesity rate climbing as high as 56 percent, lots of us are sugar addicts. Sugar can be more addictive than drugs like heroin or cocaine because sugar is a slow, silent addiction as opposed to louder, quicker drug addictions. A sugar addict doesn't get hooked right away. It could take 10 years, but once established, the addiction is just as strong, and just as dangerous. The result is obesity, diabetes, heart disease, and more.

When you are addicted to sugar, you feel moody when you don't eat it. The smell, sight, or touch of sugary foods can give you an instant high or rush, and spark a craving. And when you are not eating sugar, you're thinking about it. You literally cannot go a day without it. What's more, when you do eat sugar, you tend to eat too much.

Sugar dependency is a sign of a dopamine imbalance. Sugar and its many hidden forms—high fructose corn syrup, fructose, dextrose, sucralose, molasses, and honey—all deplete your dopamine, which will reduce your sexual desire. Like any other addiction, it can be passed down for two to three generations, so if you can break the habit when you are young, you are also protecting the lives of your children, and possibly your grandchildren. With rising childhood obesity rates, each generation seems to be getting worse—or more addicted.

A sugar addiction is difficult to avoid but easy to break. The first thing you need to do is switch to sugar substitutes. While they won't end the cravings for something sweet, they will drastically lower your caloric intake, which is the first part of the problem. Use sugar substitutes like Stevia for cooking, baking, and sweetening your coffee, other beverages, and foods.

Next, slowly decrease the amount of sugar you are using, and replace the taste with something else, like fruit or spices, which are high in nutrients. Instead of sprinkling sugar on your oatmeal or coffee, try a sprinkle of cinnamon. Instead of sweetening your tea, try adding lemon. Slowly, your tastes will change, and you'll be satisfied with a host of different flavors, from savory to spicy.

Last, you can balance your brain's chemistry to beat the sugar withdrawal. Drink lots of green tea to flush out the sugar stored in your body. You'll also be helping your body get rid of other harmful toxins and gaining nutrients.

Breaking Down Your Fat Choices

Fats are necessary for overall health and sexual health. As we discussed in Chapter 5, good fats are important to keep your acetylcholine high for smoother, gliding, and wetter sex. Choosing the best sources of choline means being picky about the types of fats you eat.

Saturated fats, which become solid at room temperature (like butter), are now on the "yes" list, but in limited quantities. In fact, a small amount of saturated fat is not unhealthy as long as it is combined with the other types of fats. I tell my patients to choose low-fat (1 percent or 2 percent) milk instead of fat free and to choose low-fat yogurt instead of fat free.

Monounsaturated fatty acids are liquid or soft at room temperature and are the best fats to choose from. They are found in foods like olive oil, avocado, nuts, seeds, and egg yolks.

Polyunsaturated fatty acids are slightly more complicated. They are also a good source of fat and are found in many plant and animal foods. There are two types of polyunsaturated fats, the omega-3's and the omega-6's. Omega-3 fats play a pivotal role in maintaining good health: They have the ability to increase blood flow so fats are more easily delivered to the sites of metabolism, where they then stimulate metabolism. And, because they can increase blood flow, they are the best fats to choose to boost your SexQ.

Unfortunately, omega-3 fats occur naturally only in a few plants, like flax, a few fish, like salmon and shrimp, and eggs from specially raised chickens. Fish oil is rich in two omega-3 polyunsaturated fatty acids called EPA and DHA and is the best source of omega-3 essential fatty acids. Cutting out saturated fats worsens your omega-3 status.

The omega-6 polyunsaturated fatty acids are found in highest quantities in vegetable oils like corn, soybean, and safflower oil. The omega-6's are also the polyunsaturated fat found in chicken, beef, and pork. Because omega-6's are found in so many of the foods we normally eat, we usually get enough of these fats to meet our dietary needs. Omega-3 fats are called essential because they have to be supplied from outside of the body. The key is to keep the ratio of 3's to 6's even, which is why you may need to focus on and probably supplement your omega-3 consumption. You'll need to take at least 3 grams of omega-3 fish oil a day to get the amount of omega-3 you'll need.

The Dairy Dilemma

Eating dairy foods is an excellent way to boost acetylcholine production, and they also contain important vitamins and minerals, like calcium. However, your need for calcium increases at the same time your ability to digest dairy decreases. Instead, choose foods that are high in calcium that are not dairy products, such as:

- Almonds
- Brazil nuts
- Collard greens
- Molasses
- Sardines
- Soy milk
- Soy nuts
- Spinach
- Tofu

EXERCISE IS ONE ROUTE TO GREAT SEX

Exercise can act as an aphrodisiac because it causes the body to release endorphins. Endorphins not only give you the feeling of a "runner's high" but may also help produce testosterone, which powers your sex drive. People who exercise regularly are more easily aroused and reach orgasm more quickly than those who don't. In a University of Vermont College of Medicine study of women ages 45 to 55, the subjects' sexual satisfaction correlated directly to their fitness level.

One reason is that physical exercise helps to balance your brain chemistry. We already knew that exercise improves almost every aspect of your health. Now the latest studies link exercise to improving your sex life as well, and I'm not just talking about Kegels. A 2009 study from the University of Groningen in the Netherlands shows that building muscle mass leads to both neurogenesis, the creation of new brain cells, and angiogenesis, the increase in the amount of blood that flows to the brain.

By creating new brain cells, we enhance brain functioning on both the physiological and the chemical level. This is one important way to reverse aging and increase hormone production in the brain and throughout the body. But when we are speaking about sex, it's also important to increase blood flow to areas that require heightened sensation. When cerebral blood volume increases, blood circulates to the rest of the body more freely, enhancing sexual pleasure. Both men and women will experience superior arousal; more blood flow to the genital areas increases your capacity for sensation and is ultimately the pleasure of sex. Women will experience better lubrication, and men will have larger erections.

When you increase your muscle mass through exercise and diet, you will not only look and feel younger because you are in better shape, but you will also begin to experience better, more energetic sex. Best of all, you'll begin to feel better about your body, so you can focus on your partner's performance instead of hiding under the covers.

I know it's hard to fit exercise into an already busy schedule, but it is doable, and it should be a mandatory part of every day. For maximum weight loss and health you need 7 hours of exercise a week. That means 1 hour of exercise a day, either all at once or broken into two or three intervals. If you can exercise while you watch television in the evening, you'll find that you have much more energy afterward, especially for sex. What's more, you'll also be staying away from unhealthy snacking.

You may even find that sex right after exercise is particularly intimate. After 35 to 40 minutes of moderate exercise, everything in your body is working toward achieving good sex: Your blood is circulating, your nervous system is firing, your joints and muscles are loose, and your mind is relaxed.

Starting an Exercise Program

While exercise should involve pushing your physical and mental limits, consistent pain should not be a part of the program. A great many of my patients who are overweight also suffer from chronic pain. If you fall into this category, make sure to discuss any new exercise program with your doctor. Make sure that you are properly assessed for underlying injuries, and go through appropriate rehab to build a bridge toward independent exercise. In my office all patients are screened by a chiropractor to assess for the correct level of entry or reentry into an exercise regimen.

The PATH to Exercise

In my office, we've created a five-phase program to introduce exercise. Each phase features a different type of exercise, and you can fill in what you like to do best that correlates with each phase. When you believe that you've mastered the phase, move on to the next. Each consecutive phase becomes more physically vigorous and challenging.

Some people find they are more successful working out at the gym, either alone or with a friend, or even a personal trainer. Others like to exercise in the privacy of their own homes. Whatever will work for you and your schedule is the best choice, as long as you keep the commitment to exercise.

Phase 1: Basic stretching and warmup shouldn't last longer than a week. Start by doing basic stretches that will help unlock tight muscles and joints. Work up to walking for 15 continuous minutes every day. Make sure that all of your stretching is completely pain free, and if you do feel pain, stop immediately and start again using less pressure.

Phase 2: Dynamic combinations of stretches induce blood flow and get your heart pumping. Yoga, Pilates, and low-intensity aerobic movements offer complex sequences of individual positions to transition you toward more vigorous exercise.

Yoga is a particularly good choice because it can help resolve specific sex problems and increase blood flow to the rest of the body. It also:

- Deepens the connection you feel with your partner (especially if you do it together)
- Improves your understanding of yourself and your partner
- Puts you in harmony with your body and mind, making you a better partner
- Allows you to loosen up so you can get into a wider variety of sexual positions

Phase 3: Aerobic/cardiovascular training requires rhythm and synchrony of whole body in various actions. Running, speed walking, swimming, tennis, and basketball are all good choices, as well as any other activity you like to participate in. Dancing is a great Phase 3 activity, especially if you do not like to exercise.

Phase 4: Weight lifting/resistance training strengthens muscles and bones. Resistance training can help you break bad habits like poor posture that have persisted for decades and that may cause injury. If you can afford it, it's well worth the money to work with a personal trainer who can teach you proper form, at least for your first few efforts.

Phase 5: Interval training is the dynamic combination of Phase 3 cardio and Phase 4 resistance to enhance hormone balance, break down scar tissue, and strengthen connective muscular tissue. It is the highest level of exercise for peak performance.

Continue to increase the difficulty level of exercise in order to keep improving your health. Interval programs that combine the two regimens help you achieve this goal while keeping your brain and body sharp.

Meet the METs

How much weight you gain or lose is largely dependent upon how much energy you expend versus the amount of energy you take in as food. The MET score is a measure of the intensity of a physical activity per hour. The list below shows the energy requirements of the most common physical activities, ranging from stagnant to vigorous exercise. One MET (short for Metabolic Equivalent) is the energy expended at rest. Two METs indicate that the energy required to perform the action is twice that used when you are at rest. Three METs is triple the resting energy expenditure, and so on. A MET-minute can be used to quantify the total amount of physical activity in a way that is comparable across different types of activities. For example, a tennis doubles game for half an hour accounts for about 100 MET-min, the equivalent of walking uphill for 10 minutes. A common guideline is that total regular physical activity must fall in the range of 500 to 1,000 MET-minutes per week to produce substantial health benefits.

Less than 3 METs:

- Light housekeeping
- Standing
- Golf (using a cart)
- Walking slowly (2 mph)
- Stationary bike

3–5 METs:

- Cleaning windows
- Raking
- Golf (walking)
- Sailing
- Tennis (doubles)
- Sex
- Light calisthenics

5–7 METs:

- Gardening
- Tennis (singles)
- Downhill skiing
- Light backpacking
- Basketball
- Stream fishing
- Level walking (4.5–5.0 mph)
- Bicycling
- Swimming (breast stroke)
- Carpentry

7–9 METs:

- Heavy shoveling (dirt or snow)
- Canoeing
- Mountain climbing
- Level jogging

Your SexQ Impacts Exercise

- A high dopamine person is drawn to variety and risk and is likely to get injured during exercise.
- The low dopamine person likes repetition and may focus on one part of the body rather than training different parts.
- High acetylcholine types will connect with team sports rather than individual training.
- Low acetylcholine types might become too specifically trained and overtrain one part of the body.
- The GABAs, feeling-oriented people, need more social connections, and they may prefer less beneficial team sports over individual sports that promote longevity, like weight lifting, running, or swimming.
- A high serotonin sex style is the typical weekend warrior who exercises for fun but lacks the consistency needed to make exercise a daily routine that yields results.
- The low serotonin person lacks feeling, so they might not sense the beginning signs of injuries or stress until too late.

- Swimming (crawl stroke)
- Rowing machine
- Heavy calisthenics

More than 9 METs:

- Climbing stairs quickly
- Squash
- Cross-country skiing
- Running
- Jumping rope
- Walking uphill

SUPPLEMENTS FOR ENHANCING EXERCISE PERFORMANCE

Choose from this list, depending on your current health issues and particular exercise goals.

- **Coenzyme Q10** leads to the production of a high-energy molecule (ATP) that may increase endurance in any kind of physical activity. Coenzyme Q10 is also an excellent fat-soluble antioxidant.
- **Creatine** is a high-energy molecule that may be of benefit during short periods of strenuous exercise.
- **Egg protein** is sold in powdered form and is another alternative for people who cannot tolerate whey (i.e., those with milk/dairy allergies).
- **Glucosamine and chondroitin** provide joint support by reducing inflammation and promoting the rebuilding of worn-out joints.
- **Glutamine** supplementation helps restore glutamine lost during intense exercise in order to build muscles. Glutamine also supports the immune system and reduces postexercise infections.
- **L-carnitine** is a vitamin-like molecule that helps to burn long-chain fatty acids (fat). It is particularly good for the heart, since the heart gets most of its fuel from fat.

- **Whey protein** is the highest-quality protein that is also easily and quickly absorbed. Although it is not as good as real protein, it contains high amounts of the branched chain amino acids (BCAA) that muscles use as an energy source, although not enough for your brain to absorb. Whey protein also contains compounds that support the immune system.

THE SEVEN SEVENS OF SEX

In order to be able to continue to have great sex and even greater intimacy, you should take your healthy lifestyle training to the next level every day and have at least:

- Seven teaspoons of different spices
- Seven servings of fruits and vegetables, as variously colored as possible
- Seven 6-ounce servings of tea, hot or cold
- Seven minutes of quiet contemplation
- Seven repetitions of your favorite strength-training exercise
- Seven hours of sleep
- Seven hugs or other expressions of emotional support and physical contact

By incorporating a life-enhancing program, you'll not only look better, but you'll feel better. When you feel good about yourself, you'll feel younger and sexier, and be better able to take care of yourself now and in the long run.

CHAPTER 13

Love Better, Live Better

BY THIS POINT you've learned many different ways to take better care of yourself, and in so doing, improve your SexQ. Hopefully you've gained new insight into the person you really are, and what you truly want your sex life to look and feel like. More important, you understand that you are not condemned to living with your current SexQ if it is not making you feel satisfied, healthy, and young. You've discovered new treatment options that can rebalance your brain and improve your sexual performance so that the years ahead of you will be just as exciting and passionate as the years behind you. And you've learned ways to change your lifestyle now, so you can continue to look and feel younger, and sexier, going forward.

Now it's time to start thinking about the other half of your sexual equation. When you've mastered your own SexQ, you may find that you are more—or less—sexually compatible with your spouse/partner. If there is some aspect of incompatibility, it's not only appropriate but necessary to investigate,

to find out why there are differences, and more important, how you can facilitate change so both of you are sexually satisfied within a loving, intimate relationship.

The state of marriage in our culture is precarious at best. I sometimes feel that there is so much stress in this world that it's causing an epidemic of brain chemical imbalances. Intimacy has become connected with naughty behavior instead of a sustained, loving relationship. If you are having trouble in your relationship, you need to think about your age, your health, and your brain, because all of these factors can sabotage your ability to relate to and love others. This is true whether you are straight, gay, or anywhere in between.

Worse, many couples find that they are bored with different aspects of their marriage, and sex is no exception. So just as you go about mixing up your weekly recipes, you have to mix up your sex life. Otherwise, you won't be able to sustain a marriage, no matter how compatible you are.

If there is only one lesson you take away

from this book, it's that your sex life is in your control. But great sex is an education in partnership and communicating. Work together to clearly identify exactly how satisfied you each feel with the state of your sexual union, and what you are willing to change. Opening the sexual dialogue is the first step to keeping your marriage fresh, forever.

Remember, sex is probably our most vulnerable state, whether it is within the confines of a committed, loving relationship or not. It can, and often does, hurt people emotionally and leave them scarred. The ideas we create about sex conjure fantasies that can never be fulfilled, even on a day-to-day basis in normal love. That's why sex needs to be accompanied by two balanced brains and two healthy bodies. If you feel that yours is now on track, it's time to work with your spouse so the two of you can continue on this sexual journey together.

The Sages on Sex

Nachmanides, also known as Ramban, was a great physician and Torah scholar of the 13th century. One of his most famous writings is the Egeret HaKodesh, or "Holy Letter," which serves as an inspirational sex and relationship manual. One of the first things that Nachmanides teaches is that it's important for every couple to communicate about desire itself. We have to be able to tell our partners what gives us pleasure and what our sexual needs might be.

He also explains that foreplay is central to the sexual act, because it displays one partner's concern for the other. The best sex occurs when neither party is rushing.

A YOUNGER (SEXIER) YOU IS VITAL FOR LONG-LASTING RELATIONSHIPS

These questions are really conversation starters to improve your SexQ as a couple.

VARIETY

- How often would I like to have sex?
- When and where do I want to have sex?
- In what positions do I want to have sex?

ROMANCE

- Am I dependent on sex toys?
- What do I need for stimulation?
- How do I define the right mood for sex?

COMMITMENT

- Do I have sexual clarity?
- Am I bisexual?
- Am I a trisexual, willing to "try anything"?

ADVENTURE

- Is sex stabilizing my relationship?
- Am I really open to change?
- Is sex really fun for me?

IS S/HE CRAZY OR JUST OLD?

People confuse sexual dysfunction with psychological issues all the time. However, I know that changes to your sexual behavior are more than likely due not to a psychological shift but are instead signs of a changing, aging brain chemistry. One should not fall into the trap of attributing sexuality entirely to emotions. When I meet new patients, my first assumption is that their complaints have a chemical basis and can be reversed to restore a more loving marriage by restoring the individual's brain chemistry.

Sexual dysfunction is not psychological, it's physical. Low arousal, low desire, and infrequent orgasm are all signs of poor brain chemistry and poor health, especially if the symptoms are new. If your spouse used to look forward to having sex with you and now seems less interested, chances are that one or both of you have experienced a change in brain chemistry. However, the good news is that by restoring two brains, you can enhance every aspect of sex to make it more enjoyable for you both. Sexually speaking, men are generally "younger" than women and desire sex more often. But women can get younger: I see it all the time.

INTIMACY MEANS DEEPLY UNDERSTANDING YOUR SPOUSE

Healthy personal relationships are much more than great sex: There should be an emotional as well as a physical connection. The results of your SexQ quiz combined with the results from the temperament

> ### HIS and HERS
> The typical man likes to feel that he is capable of having sex whenever he wants to. Women crave the emotional connection: They need to feel the love before they can be secure in themselves to ask for more.
> - Men need HIS: Happiness, Intimacy, Sex
> - Women need HERS: Happiness, Ecstasy, Romance, Sex

quiz in Chapter 3 provide detailed information that links the brain's chemistry and individual character. For example, we now know that dopamine levels determine each individual's ability to be either extroverted or introverted. Acetylcholine adjusts thinking preferences. GABA increases organizational skills. Serotonin generates feelings and motivation for pleasure-seeking and is linked to various sensing and feeling behaviors.

When each of the brain chemicals is produced at the right level, you feel powerful, calm, rested, and motivated to learn. However, when any or all are out of balance, they result in illness as well as less-than-ideal behavior patterns. Here are some clues to see if your spouse/partner is deficient in any brain chemicals. By resolving them, you will be able to regain your emotional connection.

Dopamine-Deficient Personalities

The Loner lacks the energy to socialize and has difficulty expressing their needs for sex, let alone expressing feelings of love, joy, sadness, desire, or rage. A natural remoteness can become extreme. These people are not romantic and are not interested in sexual variety. They also have a hard time understanding or appreciating the feelings of others.

The Procrastinator lacks the energy to meet their sexual needs. If angry, a procrastinator will avoid confrontation. Like loners, they also have a hard time understanding or appreciating others' feelings.

The Masochist remains in abusive relationships and can reject help to avoid being a burden. May possibly get themselves in over their heads sexually, to the point that they are in physical danger.

Acetylcholine-Deficient Personalities

The Eccentric seems odd, even bizarre. These personalities feel normal in isolated situations and steer away from human interaction. These people do not like to be touched and are not interested in sexual variety.

The Perfectionist lacks the ability to end or get off task. Has difficulty making decisions, because they are always striving for the ideal situation that never presents itself. This is not a romantic individual and can be someone who is constantly putting off sex until they are "in the mood."

The Nurturer fears being alone or abandoned, so allows others to make decisions for them. Like masochists, they may find themselves in sexually precarious situations because they are so eager to please.

GABA-Deficient Personalities

The Unstable lack control in every aspect of life, including sex. Personal care is often neglected, and a general feeling of emptiness persists as a result of loss of relationships. These people are not romantic and, sexually, can take risks or choose multiple partners in an attempt to find a relationship. They may also have obsessive-compulsive traits that delay intimacy and sexuality.

The Drama queen/king is inappropriately theatrical. This person has a wild streak and often insists on being the center of attention, constantly searching for reassurance of their worth. These types of people are likely to wander sexually.

The Painfully shy is easily hurt, so avoids social interactions and activities.

The Aggressive likes to intimidate and humiliate others, can be verbally or physically abusive. They also have a hard time understanding or appreciating others' feelings. These people are often sexually dominant and potentially dangerous unless their partners can take control.

Serotonin-Deficient Personalities

The Self-absorbed lacks sensitivity to others. Self-image is based on fantasy and exaggeration, to the point where the boundary between truth and lies is blurred. They end up depressed, lying around the house all day and checking out porn on the Internet, instead of putting in the time to develop a meaningful relationship.

The Rule breaker lacks sensitivity to society at large. They are overly impulsive and shortsighted, proceeding rashly without considering consequences.

The Suspicious easily feels slighted and is quick to counterattack. Carries grudges and bad feelings. Avoids sexual contact because they are afraid of others.

GETTING THE BIG PICTURE

While we are each dominant in one brain chemical group, we are actually a combination of each. When brain chemistry changes, it's possible to shift from one personality type to another. These shifts in biotemperaments can also occur during illness.

The following descriptions identify the 16 likely varieties of generalized biotemperaments. They are based on brain chemical combinations.

The quiz in Chapter 3 allowed you to determine your temperament. Then combine all four choices: Your particular temperament is one of 16 possible outcomes. Then do the same exercise for your spouse or partner and see if you can understand him or her a little bit better. The second table identifies the SexQ of each of these combinations. Though brief, these descriptions often get right to the essence of a person's internal motivation.

Once you understand where you and your partner are each coming from, you can create a course of action for your relationship together. The fix begins with balancing each of your brain chemistries. Your program may be quite different from that of your spouse. However, together, you will be able to reach a level of sexuality that you are both comfortable with.

PERSONALITY TYPE	DOMINANT BIOCHEMICAL
Extroversion	+ Dopamine
Introversion	− Dopamine
INtuitive	+ Acetylcholine
Sensing	− Acetylcholine
Judging	+ GABA
Perceiving	− GABA
Feeling	+ Serotonin
Thinking	− Serotonin

INJT: Tons of original ideas and great drive. Skeptical, critical, independent, determined, often stubborn.

INPT: Quiet, reserved, impersonal. Usually interested mainly in ideas, with little liking for parties or small talk. Tend to have sharply defined interests.

ENPT: Quick, ingenious, good at many things. Stimulating company, alert, and outspoken. Apt to turn to one new interest after another. Has no boundaries and assigns no feeling or attachment to sex; it's just an act.

ENJT: Hearty, frank, decisive, leaders. Are usually well-informed and enjoy adding to their fund of knowledge. May sometimes be more positive and confident in an area than their experience warrants.

INJF: Succeed by perseverance, originality, and desire to do whatever is needed or wanted. Quietly forceful, conscientious, concerned for others. Respected for their firm principles.

INPF: Full of enthusiasms and loyalties, but seldom talk of these until they know you well. Care about learning, ideas, language, and independent projects of their own. Tend to undertake too much, then somehow get it done. Friendly but often too absorbed in what they are doing to be sociable. Little concerned with possessions or physical surroundings.

ENPF: Warmly enthusiastic, high-spirited, ingenious, imaginative. Quick with a solution for any difficulty and ready to help anyone with a problem. Often rely on their ability to improvise instead of preparing in advance.

ENJF: Responsive and responsible. Generally feel real concern for what others think or want. Responsive to praise and criticism.

ISJF: Quiet, friendly, responsible, and conscientious. Work devotedly to meet their obligations. Thorough, painstaking, accurate. Loyal, considerate, concerned with how other people feel.

ISPF: Quietly friendly, sensitive, kind, modest about their abilities. Usually do not care to lead but are often loyal followers. Often relaxed about getting things done, because they enjoy the present moment and do not want to spoil it by undue haste or exertion.

ESPF: Outgoing, easygoing, accepting, friendly, enjoy everything and make things more fun for others by their enjoyment. Have sound common sense and practical ability with people as well as with things.

ESJF: Warmhearted, talkative, popular, conscientious. Need harmony and may be good at creating it. Always doing something nice for someone.

ISJT: Serious, orderly, realistic, and dependable. See to it that everything is well organized. Make up their own minds as to what should be accomplished and work toward it steadily, regardless of protests or distractions.

ISPT: Cool onlookers—quiet, reserved, observing and analyzing life with detached curiosity and unexpected flashes of original humor. Exert themselves no more than they think necessary, because any waste of energy would be inefficient.

ESPT: Matter-of-fact, do not worry or hurry, enjoy whatever comes along. May be a bit blunt or insensitive. Adaptable, tolerant, generally conservative in values.

ESJT: Practical, realistic, matter-of-fact. Like to organize and run activities. May make good administrators, especially if they remember to consider others' feelings and points of view.

THE FIVE LOVE LANGUAGES

In his best-selling book, *The Five Love Languages,* Gary Chapman, PhD, describes the five ways in which people define how they want to be loved. In order to truly bond with your spouse, you need to understand what he or she is looking for in a relationship, and how he or she is assuming that your love will be expressed. This is difficult, because many of us never bother to tell each other what our expectations are. However, it is so very

How the Brain Controls Sex

	DOPAMINE E/I*	ACETYLCHOLINE N/S*	GABA J/P*	SEROTONIN F/T*
ENJF: Balanced brain sex	high	high	high	high
ENJT: "Up for adventure" sex	high	high	high	low
ENPF: Uncontrolled romantic	high	high	low	high
ENPT: Enjoys multiple partners and/or a variety of sexual activity	high	high	low	low
ESJF: Low romance; "let's just do it"	high	low	high	high
ESJT: High sex within marriage	high	low	high	low
ESPF: Loves action and touch	high	low	low	high
ESPT: Free-loving spirit	high	low	low	low
INJF: Romantic controller	low	high	high	high
INJT: Frigid romantic	low	high	high	low
INPF: Romantic, touchy, orgasmic	low	high	low	high
INPT: Romantic dreamer	low	high	low	low
ISJF: Lover, yet dutiful sex drive	low	low	high	high
ISPF: Loves to give an orgasm: lives for the emotion around the orgasm	low	low	low	high
ISJT: Routine sexuality	low	low	high	low
ISPT: Rough-around-the-edges sex	low	low	low	low

*See key on pages 24 to 25.

important to express your heartfelt commitment in a way that your spouse will receive your message and appreciate you.

To my mind, each of Chapman's love languages can be directly related to a SexQ.

- **Words of affirmation:** Means that s/he wants to hear that they are loved and appreciated, which can be a sign of a high serotonin SexQ
- **Quality time:** Means that s/he wants to do things together, which can be a sign of an organized, high GABA SexQ
- **Receiving gifts:** Means that s/he likes to be given tokens of your affection, which means that you need to cultivate intuition, a high acetylcholine SexQ
- **Acts of service:** Means that s/he likes to be taken care of, another sign of a high GABA SexQ
- **Physical touch:** Means that s/he enjoys personal contact, a sign of a sensing, low acetylcholine SexQ

CREATING COMPATIBILITY

When a couple enhances or balances their SexQ, they are able to achieve more together than either can do alone. For example, when you enhance dopamine, your sexual relationship will be able to attain more variety. You may also notice that your communication will be clearer because you and your spouse will be more outgoing and honest with each other. With more acetylcholine, your sex life can become more creative, and you will gain deeper insight into your relationship. With more GABA, you can relax before sex and be able to see your relationship in the proper perspective. With more serotonin, sex can become much more fun, and you'll be able to tap into your deep feelings for each other.

By dialing down your brain chemistry, you'll come to have more tact and appreciation for each other. I know that, more than anything else, relationships require forethought. But when you have a high dopamine SexQ, you often say the first thing that comes into your mind, which can get you into big trouble. As my colleague Dr. Daniel Amen often says, "No forethought equals no foreplay."

Just as you can enhance or deplete your SexQ, you can also modify your character and temperament. Diet, lifestyle changes, medication, or nutrient supplements will definitely make a difference. However, you may also need to retrain your brain by purposefully changing your outlook. You can teach an old dog new tricks—particularly if you are the old dog. And you can work with your spouse/partner so that they can see the light and change their ways as well.

Those with similar SexQs ultimately get along best. Ideally, you and your partner should have three out of four temperament types in common. However, sometimes couples with brain chemistries that are too similar run into problems. For example, two high dopamine SexQs can each go in their own directions. Where there's too much variety, there's not enough continuity. Two intuitives can be ridiculously romantic and lose their connection to reality. If both you and your spouse are high GABA, then sex will quickly become too routine. And two high serotonins together can be too flaky, spending too much of their day making themselves happy without getting anything done.

The following exercises will help you develop the less dominant aspects of your brain chemistry in order to achieve a more balanced SexQ. They are meant to focus nonphysical attention on your relationship, to deepen your level of intimacy, create connectedness, and secure the bond that originally brought the two of you together.

To Increase Your Sexual Variety

Sharing: Share a private thought with someone who is not a close friend.

Processing out loud: Talk about a new idea with your spouse while you are formulating it. Share your process as it is happening, including your feelings, thoughts, desires, fantasies.

Variety: Try two or three new recreational activities with your spouse.

To Develop a More Deeply Focused Relationship

Focus: Spend at least an hour a week with your spouse outside of the bedroom and away from the television and other distractions. See if you can experience your spouse on a deeper level by relearning his or her interests outside of the family you have created.

Listening: Listen to what your partner is saying, staying attentive to them rather than formulating a response in your own mind. Give him/her the space to verbalize thoughts without interruption.

Reflection: Pause for 15 seconds before you say anything to your spouse, whether it is positive or negative. See if you can formulate your ideas before speaking; do not express the first idea that you are conscious of.

Calmness: When you experience an emotion surfacing that you do not want to share, physically remove yourself from the triggering environment. Once you are calm, return and explain to the best of your ability why you were so emotionally charged, and then work together to achieve a positive result for everyone involved.

To Develop Your Romantic, Intuitive Side

Going beyond the present: With your spouse, think of 20 different solutions to a family problem (for example, how to plan for retirement).

Connecting with the cosmos: Play a game with your spouse where you take turns saying a random word, and without thinking, responding with the first word or thought that comes to your mind.

Thinking symbolically: Look at the physical things you have collected in your life. What do they symbolize for you? For example, a sports car may say, "I am successful." Then think about what these same things mean to your spouse.

To Connect to the Here and Now and Let Go of the Past

Use of senses: Have your partner close his or her eyes. Feed him a few bites of different types of food that he has not seen. Instruct him to focus on the different tastes and textures, chewing the food slowly and thoroughly, tasting the different flavors. Reverse roles with different foods and compare results.

Being present: Take time to eat dinner with your spouse, remaining focused on conversation and being aware of what is happening at each moment.

Attention to detail: Explain to your spouse, step by step, how you accomplished something you consider to be mundane, like tying shoes or determining the evening's meal. Then, see if you can recite the details of their day.

Answer questions clearly: Practice asking questions that can only be answered with a specific response. If you get a vague response, ask the question in another way until you get a less generalized answer. For example, "What do you want to do tonight?" *"Go out for dinner."* "Where would you like to go?" *"Mario's on East Street."*

To Organize Your Life to Make Room for Sex

Structure: Examine your home with your spouse. Look at the work space, kitchen, bathroom, and bedroom. Are these spaces organized in a way that really works best? Do they meet your comfort, efficiency, and aesthetic needs?

Planning/scheduling: Discuss with your spouse your ideas for your next vacation. Together, list the activities you want to do and where you want to go. Construct a plan that allows you to do all of them. Revise your list if there are too many or too few.

To Recognize Your Partner's Needs

Spontaneity: Start a day without any set plans. Choose an activity that you and your spouse have never done, and do it together.

Store information: Spend 5 minutes reading the newspaper or gathering information on the Internet about something in the external world. Spend another 5 minutes explaining the situation to your spouse. Then ask if he or she has any questions about the discussion. This exercise helps to see what type of learner your spouse is. If he needs to see what you read, he is a visual learner, which is something you'll need to take into consideration the next time you need to share information.

To Understand the Consequences of Sex and Relationships

Discover reason using logic and precision: Create an "if then" exercise: I want X. If I get X, then I will Y. If Y, then I will Z. Continue this until you come to your basic desires. For example, I want to have sex more frequently. If I can have frequent sex, I will be more relaxed at work. If I'm relaxed at work, I will be able to focus on my tasks. If I can focus . . .

Determine the consequences: Reexamine some of your goals inside your marriage and think through to where you would be if you were to achieve them.

To Develop Feeling Skills So Your Hearts Are in It Together

Cultivating intimacy: Compliment your spouse on their personality or appearance, not an accomplishment.

Building history: Talk to your partner about an experience from the past that arouses sentimental emotions in you.

Empathy: Quietly observe your spouse for 20 minutes while he or she is going about the day. Focus on their verbal and body cues to identify what they may be feeling. Later, ask them if your hypotheses were accurate.

Clarify your relationship: Make a list of what you currently value in your relationship, ranking each from most important to least. Check off which aspects you are currently satisfied with, and then discuss with your spouse the outstanding issues and how you both can improve on them.

Great Sex Deserves Great Intimacy

A successful relationship begins with both partners knowing their strengths and limitations, their brain chemistry, and their SexQ. You also need to remember that not every day is going to be perfect. Healthy

How to Change Bad Habits

- Become aware when a habit creates pain for yourself or someone else.
- Recognize that change happens slowly: Give change time to occur.
- Enlist the support of your family and friends. Let them know your intention and ask them to gently work with you toward your new goal.
- Remove yourself from any environment that reinforces your bad habits.
- Find new activities to replace old habits.

relationships survive the ups and downs of daily living, especially when you are sexually compatible and share a distinct worldview. Hopefully, I've been able to teach you the secrets to having a more intimate, deeper-feeling relationship. I practice this every day with my own wife, by remembering this anagram:

Relationship CHAMPS Know the Following:

Compliments are always appreciated.

Honoring opinions shows respect.

Affection shows that you care.

Matched sexual parity is more fulfilling than financial riches.

Passion should exist in all aspects of your lives, not just the bedroom.

Spirituality and **S**ensitivity open the doors to let love in.

CHERISHING SEX NOW AND FOREVER

I found a wonderful piece in the *New York Times* written by a 70-year-old artist, Nancy Price Freedman, as I was writing this book. When asked at a routine doctor's visit if she and her husband were still sexually active, her impulse was to say, "None of your business!" Instead, Nancy looked him straight in the eye and said, "Yes, we are."

I'm hoping you can achieve what Nancy and her husband have. With good health and a balanced brain, there is no reason why you cannot maintain an active sex life well into old age. With a better understanding of yourself and your spouse, you will be able to maintain the intimacy that stokes the fire of passion. With that, sexual desire, arousal, and orgasm will continue to come easily. And with better sex, you will have a longer, healthier, younger life for years to come.

Acknowledgments

THE CREATION OF THIS BOOK could not have been possible without the help of many individuals. I would like to thank my agent, David Vigliano, and my successful team at Rodale, led by Pam Krauss, and my publicist, David Ratner. I would also like to thank my writer, Pam Liflander, as well as my coauthor, Ellie Capria, RPA-C, for their unique skills, insights, and attentiveness in helping to get my ideas onto these pages.

I am grateful to my colleagues Tatiana Karikh, MD, and Richard Smayda, DO, who have always been invaluable critics of my work.

I am fortunate to have a gifted team of medical and administrative personnel who have helped turn my ideas into successful work. Their skills are unsurpassed, and I am lucky to have them: Uma Damle; Victoria Gibbs; Melissa Dispensa; Anish Bajaj, DC; John Pillepich; Stanley Huang; Preeti Pusalkar; and Avani Patel.

I would also like to thank my medical staff members whose contributions to this book, as well as their loyalty and dedication to helping my patients, cannot go unnoticed: Rosina Giaccio-Williams, RPA-C, and Dallas Worth, RPA-C.

And, finally, to my patients, the greatest teachers of all, who are responsible for providing me with the material for writing this book.

God bless you all!

Resources

Amen, Daniel G. *Sex on the Brain: 12 Lessons to Enhance Your Love Life.* New York: Harmony, 2007.

Aziz, Michael. *The Perfect 10 Diet: 10 Key Hormones That Hold the Secret to Losing Weight and Feeling Great—Fast!* Naperville, IL: Source, 2010.

Chapman, Gary D. *The Five Love Languages: How to Express Heartfelt Commitment to Your Mate.* Chicago: Northfield Pub., 1995.

Goldfrank, Lewis R., and Robert S. Hoffman. *Goldfrank's Manual of Toxicologic Emergencies.* New York: McGraw-Hill, Medical Pub. Division, 2007.

Komisaruk, Barry R., Carlos Beyer, and Beverly Whipple. *The Science of Orgasm.* Baltimore: Johns Hopkins UP, 2006.

Morgenthaler, John, and Mia Simms. *The Smart Guide to Better Sex: From Andro to Zinc.* Petaluma, CA: Smart Publications, 1999.

Sadock, Benjamin J., Virginia A. Sadock, Pedro Ruiz, and Harold I. Kaplan. *Kaplan and Sadock's Comprehensive Textbook of Psychiatry.* Philadelphia: Wolters Kluwer Health/Lippincott Williams and Wilkins, 2009.

Shabsigh, Ridwan, and Bruce Scali. *Sensational Sex in 7 Easy Steps: The Proven Plan for Enhancing Your Sexual Function and Achieving Optimum Health.* New York: Rodale, 2007.

Smith, Ray B. *Cranial Electrotherapy Stimulation.* Mustang, OK: Tate, 2007.

"Normal Human Sexuality and Sexual and Gender Identity Disorders." *Diagnostic and Statistical Manual of Mental Disorders: DSM-IV-TR.* Washington, DC: American Psychiatric Association, 2000.

REFERENCES

Introduction

Knoll, J. "Sexual Performance and Longevity." *Experimental Gerontology* 32.4–5 (1997): 539–52. Print.

Chapter 1

Seldin, Daniel R., Howard S. Friedman, and Leslie R. Martin. "Sexual activity as a predictor of life-span risk." *Personality and Individual Differences* 33 (2002): 409–25. Print.

"The Medical Need for Orgasms in Women." *Foods Causing Depressions and Sleeplessness*. Web. <http://www.13.waisays.com/clitoral.htm>.

Brody, Stuart, and Tillmann H.C. Kruger. "The post-orgasmic prolactin increase following intercourse is greater than following masturbation and suggests greater satiety." *Biological Psychology* 71 (2006): 312–15. Print.

Palmore, Erdan B. "Predictors of the Longevity Difference: A 25-Year Follow-Up." *The Gerontologist* 22.6 (1982): 513–18. Print.

Smith, George Davey, Stephen Frankel, and John Yarnell. "Sex and Death: Are They Related? Findings from the Caerphilly Cohort Study." *BMJ* 315 (1997): 1641–44.

"BBC News | HEALTH | Sex Keeps You Young." *BBC News—Home*. Web. <http://news.bbc.co.uk/2/hi/health/294119.stm>.

Kary, Tiffany. "Crying Over Spilled Semen." *Psychology Today*. 1 Sept. 2002. Web. <http://www.psychologytoday.com/articles/200210/crying-over-spilled-semen>.

"Are Your Medicines Disrupting Your Sex Life?" *NetDoctor.co.uk—The UK's Leading Independent Health Website*. Web. <http://www.netdoctor.co.uk/menshealth/feature/medicinessex.htm>.

Chapter 3

Bales, K., W. Mason, C. Catana, S. Cherry, and S. Mendoza. "Neural Correlates of Pair-bonding in a Monogamous Primate." *Brain Research* 1184 (2007): 245–53. Print.

Warnock, Julia K., Anita Clayton, Harry Croft, Robert Segraves, and Faye C. Biggs. "Comparison of Androgens in Women with Hypoactive Sexual Desire Disorder: Those on Combined Oral Contraceptives (COCs) vs. Those Not on COCs." *The Journal of Sexual Medicine* 3.5 (2006): 878-82. Print.

Chapter 4

Blum, Kenneth, Amanda Chen, Thomas JH Chen, Eric R. Braverman, Jeffrey Reinking, Seth H. Blum, Kimberly Cassel, Bernard W. Downs, Roger L. Waite, Lonna Williams, Thomas J. Prihoda, Mallory M. Kerner, Tomas Palomo, David E. Comings, Howard Tung, Patrick Rhoades, and Marlene Oscar-Berman. "Activation Instead of Blocking Mesolimbic Dopaminergic Reward Circuitry Is a Preferred Modality in the Long Term Treatment of Reward Deficiency Syndrome (RDS): a Commentary." *Theoretical Biology and Medical Modelling* 5.1 (2008): 24. Print.

Blum, Kenneth, John G. Cull, Eric R. Braverman, and David E. Comings. "Reward Deficiency Syndrome." *American Scientist* 84 (1996). Print.

"Maca Restores Sexual Health without Raising Hormone Levels." *Independent News on Natural Health, Nutrition and More.* Web. <http://www.naturalnews.com/026413_maca_health_sexual_health.html>.

"Maca: Peru's Natural Viagra" *Discovery Health "Health Guides"* Web. <http://health.howstuffworks.com/sexual-health/sexual-dysfunction/maca-perus-natural-viagra.htm>.

Dording, Christina M., Lauren Fisher, George Papakostas, Amy Farabaugh, Shamsah Sonawalla, Maurizio Fava, and David Mischoulon. "A Double-Blind, Randomized, Pilot Dose-Finding Study of Maca Root (L. Meyenii) for the Management of SSRI-Induced Sexual Dysfunction." *CNS Neuroscience and Therapeutics* 14.3 (2008): 182-91. Print.

"How Maca Effects Sexual Performance of Both Men and Women." *Free Articles Directory | Submit Articles—ArticlesBase.com.* Web. <http://www.articlesbase.com/supplements-and-vitamins-articles/how-maca-effects-sexual-performance-of-both-men-and-women-736148.html>.

Geraci, Ron. "13 Ways to Naturally Boost Your Testosterone Levels." *Mens' Health* 25 Dec. 2000. Web.

Chapter 5

Walter, Chip. "Affairs of the Lips." *Scientific American* Feb.-Mar. 2008. Print.

"Hypoactive Sexual Desire Disorder in Women: Implications for Family Practice." *The Journal of Family Practice* 58.7 (2009). Print.

Nelson, Linda R., and Serdar E. Bulun. "Estrogen Production and Action." *Journal of the American Academy of Dermatology* 45.3 (2001): S116-24. Print.

Chapter 6

Dias-Ferreira, E., J. C. Sousa, I. Melo, P. Morgado, A. R. Mesquita, J. J. Cerqueira, R. M. Costa, and N. Sousa. "Chronic Stress Causes Frontostriatal Reorganization and Affects Decision-Making." *Science* 325.5940 (2009): 621-25. Print.

"GABA: Mania and Seizures to Relaxation and Impulse Control." *ENotAlone: Relationship, Personal Growth, Health Advice and Articles.* Web. <http://www.enotalone.com/article/4118.html>.

Gross A. "Sex through the ages in China." SIECUS Rep. 1981 Nov;10(2):7-8.

Chapter 7

Friedman, MD, Richard A. "Sex and Depression: In the Brain, If Not the Mind." *New York Times* [New York] 20 Jan. 2009. Print.

Aversa, A., M. Pili, D. Francomano, R. Bruzziches, E. Spera, G. La Pera, and G. Spera. "Effects of Vardenafil Administration on Intravaginal Ejaculatory Latency Time in Men with Lifelong Premature Ejaculation." *International Journal of Impotence Research* 21.4 (2009): 221-27. Print.

Shores, M. M, et al. "A Randomized, Double-blind, Placebo-controlled Study of Testosterone Treatment in Hypogonadal Older Men with Subthreshold Depression (dysthymia or minor depression)." *Journal of Clinical Psychiatry* 70.7 (2009). Print.

Chapter 8

Tural A, Yoldemir T, Erenus M. "Assessment of bone mineral density should be considered earlier in perimenopausal women with vasomotor symptoms." *Int J Gynaecol Obstet.* 2009 Nov;107(2):114-6. Epub 2009 Aug 9.

Gast GC, Grobbee DE, et al. "Vasomotor symptoms are associated with a lower bone mineral density." *Menopause.* 2009 Mar-Apr;16(2):231-8.

Sirola J, Rikkonen T. "Muscle performance after the menopause." *J Br Menopause Soc.* 2005 Jun;11(2):45-50.

Sørensen, MB. "Changes in body composition at menopause—age, lifestyle or hormone deficiency?" *J Br Menopause Soc.* 2002 Dec;8(4):137-40.

Lovejoy, JC. "The menopause and obesity." *Prim Care.* 2003 Jun;30(2):317-25.

Morisset, AS, Lemieux, S, et al. "Impact of a lignan-rich diet on adiposity and insulin sensitivity in post-menopausal women." *Br J Nutr.* 2009 Jul;102(2):195-200.

Maric, C, Sullivan, S. "Estrogens and the diabetic kidney." *Gend Med.* 2008;5 Suppl A:S103-13.

Maric, C. "Sex, diabetes and the kidney." *Am J Physiol Renal Physiol.* 2009 Apr;296(4):F680-8. Epub 2009 Jan 14.

Ainslie, DA, Morris, MJ, et al. "Estrogen deficiency causes central leptin insensitivity and increased hypothalamic neuropeptide Y." *Int J Obes Relat Metab Disord*. 2001 Nov;25(11):1680-8.

Flores-Ramos, M, Heinze, G, et al. "Association between depressive symptoms and reproductive variables in a group of perimenopausal women attending a menopause clinic in México City." *Arch Womens Ment Health*. 2009 Sep 4.

Joffe, H, Hall, JE, et al. "Vasomotor symptoms are associated with depression in perimenopausal women seeking primary care." *Menopause*. 2002 Nov-Dec;9(6):392-8.

Polisseni, AF, de Araújo, DA, et al. "Depression and anxiety in menopausal women: associated factors." *Rev Bras Ginecol Obstet*. 2009 Mar;31(3):117-23.

Braverman, ER, Chen, TJ, et al. "Preliminary investigation of plasma levels of sex hormones and human growth factor(s), and P300 latency as correlates to cognitive decline as a function of gender." *BMC Res Notes*. 2009 Jul 7;2:126.

Braverman, ER, Chen, TJ, et al. "Age-related increases in parathyroid hormone may be antecedent to both osteoporosis and dementia." *BMC Endocr Disord*. 2009 Oct 13;9(1):21.

Fantidis, P. "The role of the Stress-Related Anti-Inflammatory Hormones ACTH and Cortisol in Atherosclerosis." *Curr Vasc Pharmacol*. 2010 Jan 1.

Sephton, SE, Dhabhar, FS, et al. "Depression, cortisol, and suppressed cell-mediated immunity in metastatic breast cancer." *Brain Behav Immun*. 2009 Nov;23(8):1148-55. Epub 2009 Jul 28.

Resnick, SM, Espeland, MA, Jaramillo, SA, Hirsch, C, Stefanick, ML, Murray, AM, Ockene, J, Davatzikos, C. "Postmenopausal hormone therapy and regional brain volumes: The WHIMS-MRI Study." *Neurology*. 2009; 72; 135-142.

Coker, LH, Hogan, PE, Bryan, NR, Kuller, LH, Margolis, KL, Betterman, K, Wallace, RB, Lao, Z, Freeman, R, Stefanick, ML, Shumaker, SA. "Postmenopausal hormone therapy and sub-clinical cerebrovascular disease: The WHIMS-MRI Study." *Neurology*. 2009; 72; 125-34.

Sowers, MR, Zheng, H, McConnell, D, Nan, B, Harlow, S, Randolph, Jr., JF. "Follicle Stimulating Hormone and Its Rate of Change in Defining Menopause Transition Stages." *Journal of Clinical Endocrinology and Metabolism*. 2008; 93; 3958-64.

Jorgensen, JO, Christensen, JJ, Krag, M, Fisker, S, Ovesen, P, Christiansen, JS. "Serum insulin-like growth factor I levels in growth hormone-deficient adults: influence of sex steroids." *Hormone Research*. 2004.

Jorgensen, JO, Christensen, JJ, Vestergaard, E, Fisker, S, Ovesen, P, Christiansen, JS. "Serum insulin-like growth factor I levels in growth hormone-deficient adults: influence of sex steroids." *Hormone Research*. 2004.

Selvamani, A, Sohrabji, F. "Insulin-Like Growth Factor-1 Replacement Attenuates Estrogen-Mediated Neurotoxicity in Reproductively Aged Female Rats Following Middle Cerebral

Artery Occlusion." *The Endocrine Society.* Poster Session: Regulation and Effects of Hypothalmic Neuropeptides.

Chae, HW, Lee, EB, Kim, HS, Kim, DH. "Serum IGF-1 Increment after a Month of Growth Hormone Treatment is Effective for Prediction of Growth Response in Idiopathic Short Stature." *The Endocrine Society.* Poster Session: Growth Hormone Treatment.

Fritton, JC, Kawashima, Y, Sun, H, Mejia, W, Wu, Y, Rosen, CJ, Panus, D, Bouxsein, ML, Majeska, RJ, Schaffler, MB, Yakar, S. "Growth Hormone Protects Against Ovariectomy-Induced Bone Loss in States of Low Circulating Insulin-Like Growth Factor-1." *The Endocrine Society.* Poster Session: Insulin Like Growth Factor Signaling.

Friedrich, N, Haring, R, Nauch, M, Ludermann, J, Rosskopf, D, Spilcke-Liss, E, Felix, SB, Dorr, M, Brabant, G, Volzke, H, Wallaschofski, H. "Mortality and Serum Insulin-Like Growth Factor (IGF)-1 and IGF Binding Protein 3 Concentrations." *Journal of Clinical Endocrinology and Metabolism* 94 (5) (2009): 1732-39.

Popat, VB, Calis, KA, Vanderhoof, VH, Cizza, G, Reynolds, JC, Sebring, N, Troendle, JF, Nelson, LM. "Bone Mineral Density in Estrogen-Deficient Young Women." *Journal of Clinical Endocrinology and Metabolism* 94(7) (2009): 2277-83.

Hazzard, T.M. et al. "Down regulation of oxytocin receptors and secretion of prostaglandin F2alpha after chronic treatment of ewes with estradiol-17beta." *Biol. Reprod.* 1997 56 (6):1576-81.

Silber, M. et al. "The effect of oral contraceptive pills on levels of oxytocin in plasma and on cognitive functions." *Contraception* 1987 36 (6):641-50.

Nappi, Rossella E., and Michèle Lachowsky. "Menopause and Sexuality: Prevalence of Symptoms and Impact on Quality of Life." *Maturitas* 63.2 (2009): 138-41. Print.

Hazzard, W. R. "Atherogenesis: Why Women Live Longer than Men." *Geriatrics* 40.1 (1985). Print.

Hazzard, W. R. "Why Do Women Live Longer than Men? Biologic Differences That Influence Longevity." *Postgrad Medicine* 85.5 (1989). Print.

Vina, J. "Why Females Live Longer Than Males: Control of Longevity by Sex Hormones." *Science of Aging Knowledge Environment* 2005.23 (2005): Pe17. Print.

Franco, C., B. Andersson, L. Lonn, B.-A. Bengtsson, J. Svensson, and G. Johannsson. "Growth Hormone Reduces Inflammation in Postmenopausal Women with Abdominal Obesity: A 12-Month, Randomized, Placebo-Controlled Trial." *Journal of Clinical Endocrinology and Metabolism* 92.7 (2007): 2644-47. Print.

Chapter 9

Cawthon, PM, Ensrud, KE, Laughlin, GA, Cauley, JA, Dam, TT, Barrett-Connor, E, Fink, HA, Hoffman, AR, Lau, E, Lane, NE, Stefanick, ML, Cummings, SR, Orwoll, ES. "Osteoporotic

Fractures in Men (MrOS) Research Group. Sex hormones and frailty in older men: the osteo-porotic fractures in men (MrOS) study." *J Clin Endocrinol Metab.* 2009 Oct;94(10):3806-15. Epub 2009 Sep 8.

Baloh, RW. "Hearing and Equilibrium." In: Goldman, L, Aussiello, D, eds. *Cecil Medicine.* 23rd ed. Philadelphia, PA: Saunders Elsevier, 2007: chap 454.

Wrightson, AS. "Universal newborn hearing screening." *Am Fam Physician.* Denver, Colorado. 2007; 75(9): 1349.

Surow, Jason B. "Now Hear This: iPods May Cause Hearing Loss." 2009. *Ent and Allergy Magazine:* Volume I Issue V. <http://www.entandallergy.com/media/pdfs/enta_mag_1_v.pdf>.

Centers for Disease Control and Prevention (CDC). "Early Hearing Detection & Intervention Program." May 9, 2007.

"Hearing Impairment." March of Dimes Quick References and Fact Sheet. <http://marchofdimes. com/printablearticles/14332_1232.asp>.

Minton, B. "Aldosterone Provides New Treatment for Age-Related Hearing Loss." *Natural News.* April 2009. <http://www.naturalnews.com/026096_hearing_loss_sodium_aging.html>.

Wilson, N. "Link between Hearing Loss and lower Levels of Aldosterone Hormone." Best Syndi-cation (2006). <http://www.bestsyndication.com/Articles/2006/Nicole-WILSON/ Health/02/021006-hearing_loss_aldosterone_levels.htm>.

Bauman, PhD, N. "Aldosterone—A new treatment for hearing loss and Meniere's Disease?" Hear-ing Loss Help. March 2008. <http://hearinglosshelp.com/weblog/?p=282>.

Landau, E. "Men, convertible drivers at higher risk for hearing loss." CNN. October 2009.

Travison, T. G., A. B. Araujo, A. B. O'Donnell, V. Kupelian, and J. B. McKinlay. "A Population-Level Decline in Serum Testosterone Levels in American Men." *Journal of Clinical Endocrinology and Metabolism* 92.1 (2006): 196-202. Print.

Eure, MD, Gregg R. "Making the Best Choice." *Healthy Aging* Jan.-Feb. 2006. Print.

Howard, E. W., M.-T. Ling, C. W. Chua, H. W. Cheung, X. Wang, and Y. C. Wong. "Garlic-Derived S-allylmercaptocysteine Is a Novel In Vivo Antimetastatic Agent for Androgen-Independent Prostate Cancer." *Clinical Cancer Research* 13.6 (2007): 1847-856. Print.

Chapter 10

Byard, MD, Mark. "There's No Age Limit for Healthy Sexuality." *Journal of Longevity.* Print.

Haas, Robert. "A Natural Approach to Erectile Dysfunction That Improves Vascular Health." *Life Extension* Nov. 2009. Print.

Chapter 12

Brody, S. "Slimness is associated with greater intercourse and lesser masturbation frequency." *Journal of Sex and Marital Therapy* 30 (2004): 251–61.

Hughes, S. M., and Gallup, G. G. "Sex differences in morphological predictors of sexual behavior: Shoulder to hip and waist to hip ratios." *Evolution and Human Behavior* 24 (2003): 173–78.

Exton, M.S., T.H. Kruger, M. Koch, E. Paulson, W. Knapp, U. Hartmann, U. and M. Schedlowski. "Coitus-induced orgasm stimulates prolactin secretion in healthy subjects." *Psychoneuroendocrinology* 26(2001): 287–94.

Lindsay, David G., and Sian B. Astley. "European Research on the Functional Effects of Dietary Antioxidants." *Molecular Aspects of Medicine* 23 (2002). Print.

Rolls, Barbara J., Julia A. Ello-Martin, and Beth Carlton Tohill. "What Can Intervention Studies Tell Us about the Relationship between Fruit and Vegetable Consumption and Weight Management?" *Nutrition Reviews* 62.1 (2004): 1-17. Print.

INDEX

Underscored page references indicate sidebars and tables.

A